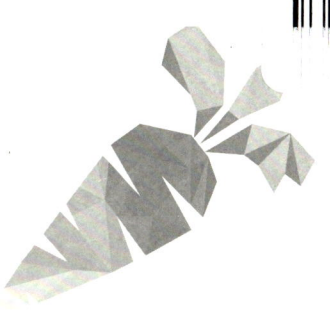

Nutrition & Weight Management Sidekick
Journal

Rewire Your Eating Habits.
Boost Health & Energy.

Created with love by
Amir Atighehchi, Ari Banayan, & Mikey Ahdoot

Copyright ©2019 Every Damn Day, LLC
All rights reserved.
Published by Every Damn Day, LLC.

No part of this publication may be reproduced, or stored in a retrieval system, or transmitted in any form or by any means, electronic, mechanical, recording, photocopying, scanning or otherwise, without express written permission of the publisher.

For information about permission to reproduce elections from this book, email team@habitnest.com
Visit our website at www.HabitNest.com

PUBLISHER'S DISCLAIMER

While the publisher and author have used their best efforts in preparing this book, they make no representations or warranties with respect to the accuracy or completeness of the contents of this book. The advice and strategies contained herein may not be suitable for your situation. You should consult with a professional where appropriate. Neither the publisher nor the author shall be liable for any loss of profit or any other commercial damages, including but not limited to special, incidental, consequential, or other damages.

The company, product, and service names used in this book are for identification purposes only. All trademarks and registered trademarks are the property of their respective owners.

SPECIAL THANKS

We'd like to extend a wholehearted, sincere thank you to Skyler Wolpert and Lindsay McDermott for formatting + editing help.
We love ya!

ISBN (Pear Green): 97809986561-6

THIRD EDITION

Information Disclaimer

The information provided by Habit Nest™ (and habitnest.com) is for educational and entertainment purposes only, and is not to be interpreted as a recommendation for a specific treatment plan, product, or course of action. Habit Nest™ does not provide specific medical advice, and is not engaged in providing medical services. Habit Nest™ does not replace consultation with a qualified health or medical professional who sees you in person, for the health and medical needs of yourself or a loved one. In addition, while Habit Nest™ frequently updates contents, medical, health and fitness information changes rapidly, and therefore, some information may be out of date. Please see a physician or health professional immediately if you suspect you may be ill or injured.

Every person has very different dietary needs based on many factors. We recommend consulting your doctor and/or nutritionist in detail before taking action on any of the information in this book.

Our Mission

We are a team of people **obsessed with taking ACTION** and **learning new things** as quickly as possible.

We love finding the **fastest, most effective ways** to build a new skill, then **systemizing that process for others**.

With building new habits, we empathize with others every step of the way *because we go through the same process ourselves*. We live and breathe everything in our company.

We use our hard-earned intuition to outline **beautifully designed, intuitive products** to help people live **happier, more fulfilled lives**.

Everything we create comes with a mix of **bite-sized information, strategy, and accountability**. This hands you a simple yet **drastically effective roadmap** to build **any skill** or habit with.

We take this a step further by diving into **published scientific studies**, the opinions of subject-matter **experts**, and the **feedback we get from customers** to further enhance all the products we create.

Ultimately, Habit Nest is a **practical, action-oriented startup** aimed at helping others take back decisional authority over every action they take. We're here to help people live **wholesome, rewarding lives** at the **brink of their potential!**

– Amir Atighehchi, Ari Banayan, & Mikey Ahdoot
Cofounders of Habit Nest

Table of Contents

1 The "Why"
- Understanding Your Why

11 The "What"
- The Science Behind Fat Loss
- Figuring out Your Macronutrient Intake
- The Phases of Building a New Habit
- Daily Content & Tracking

63 The "How"
- Perfectionists, Tread Lightly
- Important Notes on Mentality
- Sample Journal Page
- Commit

76 Phase I (Days 1-7)

96 Phase II (Days 8-21)

132 Phase III (Days 22-66)

235 Fin
- So… What Now?
- What Life Changing Habit Will YOU Conquer Next?
- Share the Love
- Meet the Habit Nest Team
- Get Daily Motivation & Guidance
- Context Index
- How Was This Journal Created?

The "Why"

Understanding Your Why

The absolute most important aspect of changing your life for the better is… **Establishing your clear, unwavering purpose (your *Why*)**.

The thing is, when we forget (and we forget quite often) the reason we're struggling to improve our lives, we tend to retreat to our habitual selves; to the person we were before we made the decision to change.

Having a clear understanding of your 'why' (what you want to change and why you want to change it) is what pulls you through the tough times you will inevitably face when altering your habits.

Here are a few simple questions that **you should take your time to answer sincerely before moving on**.

These questions are aimed at getting to the root of what drives you; finding your greatest motivation for beginning a lifestyle of health, weight loss and attainment of your goal body.

If you're going to even make an attempt at this, you better know why you're doing it in the first place.

Seriously. Take the time to get extremely clear on your Why.

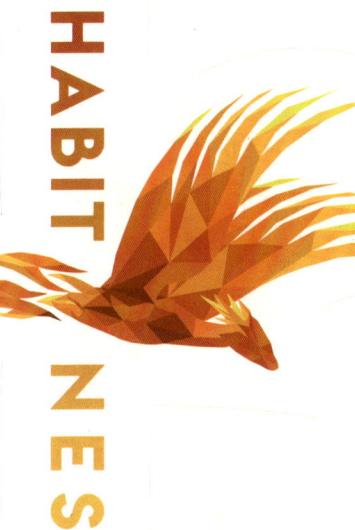

1. What would my life look like if I incorporated healthy eating into my life for the next 30 days?

_____
_____
_____
_____
_____
_____

2. What sort of ripple effect would better eating habits have on other areas of my life? On the lives of people around me?

_____
_____
_____
_____
_____
_____

3. What would my life look like if I do not do this? What would I be missing out on? How would missing those make me feel?

_____
_____
_____

_____
_____
_____
_____

Bonus Question: What are the top hurdles I'm facing with sticking to a healthy eating regimen and achieving my goal body? What do I need to do to overcome these?

_____
_____
_____
_____
_____

Bookmark this section and flip back here the next time you're struggling to stay consistent with this habit.

This section is your SOS Lifeline.

Preparing For 'Off' Days

One very valuable skill you can build is the ability to shift from having 'off' days to getting back on track with your goals. Building this skill will allow you to always be able to get back on track, no matter how far off you go, or how often.

Instead of focusing on "being perfect all the time," let's prepare for those days where, for whatever reason, something goes astray in your plans. Even the most fit, healthy people in the world have days like this. What sets them apart is their ability to deal with them.

Try to envision what an 'off day' looks like for you and what caused it. Did you not get enough sleep and can't think straight? Are you dealing with a lot emotionally and can't bring yourself to stay consistent? Are you having major food cravings and wanting to binge eat?

Don't just think about it, try to actually empathize with yourself on that day so you can be emotionally ready.

Some small actions I can take to improve my 'off' days are:

_____

_____

_____

_____

_____

_____

Before We Get Started

Please take a moment to read this because there are two things you need to understand.

1. **With this journal, you are not starting a "diet" in the way that term is ordinarily used,**

AND

2. **Everybody responds somewhat differently to food.**

   First, when we say the word 'diet,' we usually refer to a short-term method for achieving a certain amount of weight loss. Any time you see the word 'diet' in this journal, we're referring to the way you eat in general; not a quick weight loss method.

Although you can use this journal to help you achieve short-term weight loss by keeping you on track, that is not our goal for you.

We hope to help you build a lifelong habit of healthy eating so that:

1. You're maximizing your energy levels through the food you eat.
2. You're enjoying everlasting confidence by looking as good as you've always dreamed.
3. That you do it all on a consistent basis while enjoying your favorite foods.

The way this journal will guide you to add a habit of lifelong healthy eating is by:

1. Giving you a fundamental understanding of the science behind how our bodies respond to different types of food,

2. Helping you understand how you can manipulate your body to manage your weight,

3. Giving you the perfect starting point by creating a macronutrient ratio that serves your goals,

4. Thoroughly explaining the habit-building process, and

5. Providing all the accountability, motivation and information you need to follow through.

Secondly, although there are general rules that apply to healthy eating and fat loss, we all respond differently to food. The information you're getting here is accurate, but it **does not apply equally to everybody.**

The only way we can we can help you create a sustainable, healthy eating regimen that conforms to your body goals and overall life plan is if you understand the fact that you are going to go through a long learning curve in understanding the way you personally respond to changes in your diet.

You're going to have to experiment with different large-scale diets and tweak them based on information you gather about your own body.

We're here to help you start the process, make the necessary changes, and stay consistent and happy while going through it.

This breaks through the standard knowledge of "incredible wonder-diets" because those only work for a small subset of people, and many of them only work in the short-term.

By experimenting with different kinds of foods and small shifts in the foods you eat, you'll be able to see first-hand how it affects you daily.

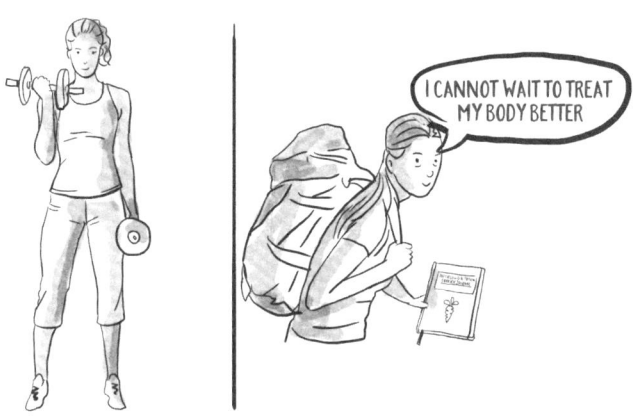

The "What"

The Science Behind Fat Loss

This guide is going to be short and sweet.

We're talking about food and the body. More specifically, we'll dig in to how to maximize your fat loss while maintaining an overall aim of health and looking the best you possibly can.

This journal's goal is to give you all the knowledge, motivation, and resources you need to create the perfect eating plan that conforms to your body type.

Everything you're about to read is backed by basic science.

There is absolutely no vague "fluff." Every single word in this intro guide serves a purpose.

We'll start with a quick explanation of your basic machinery – this physical body you possess – and the way it generally functions with regards to the intake of food.

The objective is to focus your attention in a very specific manner to establish your mindset from the right point of reference.

You Can't Lie to Your Body

As a concept, weight loss isn't difficult to understand. To lose weight, we need to burn more energy (calories) than we eat.

What most people never fully grasp, realize, or remember is that **our bodies are machines.**

Machines have a few main characteristics:

1. They respond in a unique way to external stimuli.
2. They need fuel to function properly and efficiently.
3. Maintenance is required to prevent degeneration.
4. They have many component parts, each with a definite function or "job."
5. They are predictable.
6. They can be manipulated to achieve desired results within their capabilities.

Think about your car. You buy a car because you have a need for a method of transportation – a way to get around. The car serves this overall purpose of taking you from place to place.

But a car isn't merely a mobility device. It has many parts which each play a role in creating the possibility of being your modern-day horse. In the ignition system alone, there are spark plugs, ignition wire, coil and a distributor that control the timing and flow of electricity to the engine's cylinders…

Every week or so, you need to get gas for the car, right? Every few months or year, your car needs to be serviced.

If you want your car to be louder or faster, what do you do? You get someone to alter the exhaust system, or you buy parts or subtract parts to increase all around power and torque.

You have a result you want to achieve, and you simply alter the machine to conform to your vision.

But you can't lie to your car. You can't tell it that you're giving it oil and give it orange juice instead.

The beauty of the human body is that it is a wonderfully intricate machine that responds mechanically to the appearance of new external stimuli, and it can be manipulated to achieve desired results the same exact way you can change the way a computer or car operates.

You can cause your body to respond with illness by smoking. You can cause your body to exert extreme energy with certain foods.

You can force your body to burn excess fat it holds by monitoring your macronutrient intake and obtaining the proper balance of nutrients.

But you can't tell your body to respond differently than what you put in it.

Remember every day, every meal, every moment: *You cannot lie to your body.*

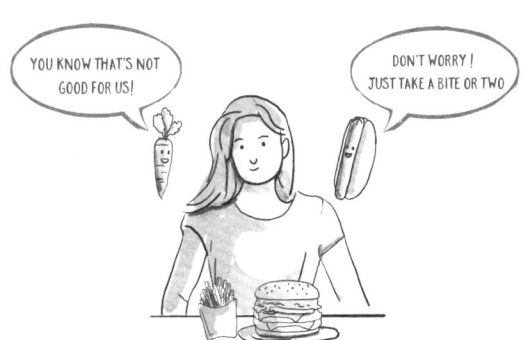

Caloric Deficit & Macronutrient Ratios

The following is assuming that your body composition goals are to:

1. Have minimal excess body fat, and
2. Maintain or increase your body's muscle

Depending on the body you want, a proper balance needs to be struck between minimizing body fat and maintaining or increasing muscle. The food we eat is the single most important factor in both decreasing body fat and improving muscle definition.

Fat Loss vs. Weight Loss

Most people don't even scratch the surface when it comes to understanding what it means to "lose weight." Weight loss can come in a few different ways.

The loss of weight that shows up on a scale can either be the result of fat loss, muscle loss, or water loss.

We all have this goal of getting to an ideal weight we think will make us happy with our physique. But the number on the scale should be the least of your worries. The goal is always to be as fit as possible, be as healthy as possible, and most importantly, to be genuinely happy with your body just as it is.

The goal is to selectively manipulate the body to burn as much fat as possible, while retaining all the muscle we have on our bodies.

An example of the distinction between fat loss and weight loss is the very well-known "no-carb" diet - complete elimination of all carbs from one's diet.

If you've heard people saying they're on a "low-carb" or "no-carb" diet that is working extremely well for them and quickly, here's why:

Every stored carbohydrate in your body holds 2.7 grams of water. Eliminating or seriously depriving your body of carbohydrates means you're losing a lot of water weight, which is good if you're looking to just drop the number on the scale quickly, but doesn't make sense if you want to achieve long-term weight loss and prevent future weight ain.

There will always be people who make it work with any diet, but drastically lowering carbs for years on end isn't realistic for most people.

Achieving a Caloric Deficit

It's simple.

Your body needs a certain amount of energy to function.

A *calorie* is a unit of energy – it is the energy value of food.

When your body uses more calories than are coming in, it is forced to turn to other places to supply and fulfill the energy requirements it isn't getting from the food you're eating.

But the body has a few options for where it can go to take the energy that it needs. It can either go to fat stores, muscle protein, or a combination of both.

Our goal in achieving fat loss is to cause the body to undergo this process of finding alternate energy supplies, while doing all that we can to force the use of fat, rather than muscle, as the primary energy source.

When there is a caloric deficit and the body is forced to turn to alternate sources of energy, it is imperative to ensure that muscle catabolism doesn't occur.

Muscle catabolism is the breakdown of muscle tissue to supply energy for the body that isn't coming from the food we're eating. This is one of the main reasons people aren't necessarily happy with their bodies when they completely cut their carbohydrate intake.

To put everything into perspective, the moment you have a caloric surplus (you eat more calories than you burn), extra calories are stored as fat for future energy use in the event that it becomes necessary.

Macronutrient Ratios

To lose weight, you need to eat less calories than you burn.[1] But the name of the game when it comes to achieving FAT loss and preventing fat gain, is **understanding how the macronutrients you eat affect the body.**

---

[1] https://sciencebasedmedicine.org/calories-in-calories-out/

Regardless of the extent of your caloric deficit, if your body isn't getting what it needs to function the way it was designed to operate, you will not be satisfied with the way you look. Instead, you will re-gain all the weight you lost the moment you start to eat like a human being.

The term **macronutrient** refers to the main types of food – carbohydrates, lipids (fats) and proteins.

The macronutrient ratio concerns the percentage of your caloric intake each of these three types of foods comprises.

To attain the right balance that will force your body to use fat for energy while retaining muscle, the macronutrient intake has to be carefully plotted and it must be tailored to your specific body type, the speed of your metabolism, and your ordinary activity levels.

In Summary:

1. Your body needs energy to function, and is in a constant state of energy expenditure.
2. A calorie is a unit of stored energy in food.
3. You can force your body to burn fat by achieving a caloric deficit.
4. A caloric deficit results where you burn more calories than you consume.
5. A caloric deficit may result in your body using muscle tissue for energy, which we can prevent with a proper balance of macronutrients.

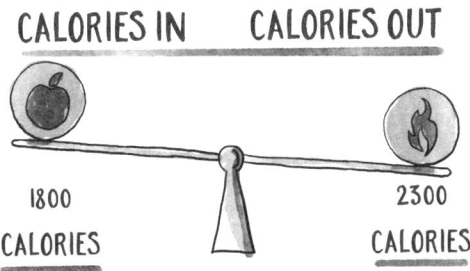

Carbohydrates

A Double-Edged Sword

We need energy to live. We need energy to breathe, to digest, to circulate blood flow, to move our limbs, to think, etc. From the moment we're born until the moment we leave this beautiful world, we are using energy to facilitate our every physical movement, thought, emotion and instinctive process.

Fat loss is really about redirecting the source of that energy by manipulating the body through the foods we eat.

The body is extremely efficient. We have a very specific process for the way we create energy based on the food we eat. When there's an excess of what is needed, the body stores it to be used in a later day.

By the same token, when there's not enough energy supply, the body adapts and finds other sources.

Carbohydrates are the body's preferred source of energy.

Carbohydrates are vital to the functioning of our bodily systems. Carbs are broken down into glucose in the body. *Glucose* is the primary molecule that serves as energy for animals like us.

We mentioned above that the main objective in achieving fat loss is forcing your body to react to circumstances you create by **using fat for energy rather than carbohydrates or muscle** tissue. We want our bodies to metabolize the fat that has been stored.[2]

That happens when the body realizes that it needs more glucose than is currently being manufactured based on the carbohydrates available, and it then releases the hormone **glucagon**, whose job is to convert existing fat that has been stored in the body into energy the body can use.

The manner in which the body responds to energy deficiencies that result from a caloric deficit is precisely dependent on how much **glycogen** your body has at any given time.

Glycogen refers to carbs that have been stored in the body. If you're continually eating carbs, which is the favored energy source, your body has absolutely no reason to metabolize fat for energy!

What's more is that when you eat more carbs than your body needs, the excess carbohydrates that can't currently be used as energy **are stored as fat**[3] so that they can potentially be used down the line if it becomes necessary.

A big part of fat loss is about regulating your carbohydrate intake to cause this bodily reaction of using fat as a source of energy. But eliminating carbs completely is the wrong way to approach the task. Although it will help you achieve weight loss, you need to make sure your body isn't forced to reach for muscle tissue as the alternate supply of energy.

---

[2] https://www.webmd.com/diabetes/type-1-diabetes-guide/what-is-ketosis#1

[3] https://www.ncsf.org/enew/articles/articles-convertingcarbs.aspx

Carbohydrates are truly a double-edged sword.

Although eliminating carbs does lead to the use of fat and muscle as alternate energy supplies, the **ingestion of carbs protects muscle tissue**, thereby forcing the burning of fat rather than muscle.[4]

*The balance is a **real** struggle:*

Too many carbs and your body won't burn fat. Too little carbs, and your body burns through your muscle tissue. But, don't worry. Soon you'll have everything you need to find the right balance for your body.

Quality of Carbs

There are two main types of carbohydrates, commonly referred to as "**simple carbs**" and "**complex carbs.**" What defines the quality of a carbohydrate is the speed at which it is absorbed – the rate at which your body breaks them down for use as energy.

Simple Carbohydrates

When carbohydrates are absorbed quickly (when simple carbohydrates are consumed), there is a quick bodily reaction of elevated blood sugar, which causes the brain to release the hormone **insulin** to get the body's blood sugar levels back under control.

---

[4] https://www.ncbi.nlm.nih.gov/pmc/articles/PMC1373635/

The resulting danger is that when insulin is set in motion to regulate blood sugar, the hormone glucagon (the hormone that asks the body to use fat as an energy supply) is halted until the insulin has finished its work. Your body regulates the blood sugar while fat burning is suppressed.

Another common negative attribute of "simple" or *fast-absorbing carbohydrates* is that giving your body that high elevation in blood sugar results in an equally low swing in the opposite direction. Basically, after insulin kicks in and lowers your blood sugar, then your body craves food to push it back up.

You feel hungry quickly.

The long-term result is a complete loss of control in the way we handle our food. We over-eat and we crave the same unhealthy carbohydrates that gave us the rush in the first place.

Regulating your carbohydrate intake is largely about regulating blood sugar levels to keep them at a balanced level.

Some examples of simple carbohydrates are: Baked goods, cookies, sugar, cereal, corn syrup, fruit juice concentrate, and dairy products.

Complex Carbohydrates

Complex carbohydrates are those that cause smaller increases in blood sugar because they take more time for the body to break down and use (they have longer chains of sugar molecules). They allow glucose to release into the bloodstream slowly and consistently.

You want to fill up your carbohydrate intake with as many complex carbohydrates as possible.

Some great complex carbs are brown rice, whole wheat bread, yams, broccoli, carrots, pasta, grains, beans, and fiber rich fruits.

Fiber is an interesting complex carbohydrate worth noting because it slows down the rate at which your body absorbs other types of carbohydrates. Fiber is also indigestible, meaning that your body completely gets rid of it after it has been made proper use of.

The Glycemic Index

The glycemic index is a scale that rates foods that can be categorized as carbohydrates based on the effect in the rise of blood sugar the food has. Generally speaking, the higher the glycemic index rating, the more "simple" the carbohydrate is.

To get the most out of the carbohydrates you consume, try checking where the carbs you eat fall on this scale. The goal is to eat foods that fall ideally from 1-40 on the scale the majority of the time, and 40-75 sparingly.

GLYCEMIC INDEX CHART
LOW GLYCEMIC (55 OR BELOW) HIGH GLYCEMIC (70 OR HIGHER)

SNACKS	G.I.	STARCH	G.I.	VEGETABLES	G.I.	FRUITS	G.I.	DAIRY	G.I.
PIZZA	33	BAGEL, PLAIN	33	BROCCOLI	10	CHERRIES	22	YOGURT, PLAIN	14
CHOCOLATE BAR	49	WHITE RICE	38	PEPPER	10	APPLE	38	YOGURT, LOW FAT	14
POUND CAKE	54	WHITE SPAGHETTI	38	LETTUCE	10	ORANGE	43	WHOLE MILK	30
POPCORN	55	SWEET POTATO	44	MUSHROOMS	10	GRAPES	46	SOY MILK	31
ENERGY BAR	58	WHITE BREAD	49	ONIONS	10	KIWI	52	SKIM MILK	32
SODA	72	BROWN RICE	55	GREEN PEAS	48	BANANA	56	CHOCOLATE MILK	35
DOUGHNUT	76	PANCAKES	67	CARROTS	49	PINEAPPLE	66	YOGURT, FRUIT	36
JELLY BEANS	80	WHEAT BREAD	80	BEETS	64	WATERMELON	72	CUSTARD	43
PRETZELS	83	BAKED POTATO	85			DATES	103	ICE CREAM	60

In Summary:

1. Eliminating carbs is not the answer to a great body, although it can help you achieve rapid weight loss.

2. The body prefers carbohydrates as its main source of energy. Carbohydrates are converted into glucose and used as energy for bodily functions and processes.

3. You can cause your body to use fat and protein as a source of energy by regulating your carbohydrate intake.

4. Carbohydrates protect your muscle tissue from being used as energy, so it is important to find the right portion of carbohydrates to eat.

5. Simple carbohydrates cause rapid increases in blood sugar, which stops your body from burning fat and leaves you feeling hungry.

6. Fill your carbohydrate intake with complex carbohydrates like yams, brown rice, whole wheat bread, grains, vegetables, quinoa, fiber-rich fruits, and beans.

7. The glycemic index rates the complexity of carbohydrates based on the way they affect blood sugar levels after consumption.

8. The lower on the glycemic index scale a carbohydrate falls, the better it is for fat loss.

Proteins

You have over 10,000 different proteins in your body. It is absolutely essential to every cell in the body. Protein is made up of amino acids, which in relation to weight loss, are important in that they **grow and repair our muscle tissue**.

It is essential to consume enough protein because it helps keep you full, stimulates muscle growth, facilitates muscle retention, and it has a significant effect on our basal metabolic rate – the automatic functioning of our metabolism.[5] The mechanics of the way protein affects the metabolism are relatively simple.

The **more protein you eat**, the **faster your metabolism works**. The faster your metabolism works, the **more calories you naturally burn**.

When paired with exercise, protein enlarges muscles by adding additional proteins to muscle fibers. The muscle-enlargement process requires amino acids. Protein is made up of amino acids and when you eat more amino acids, it has a direct effect on muscle mass.

Increasing your muscle mass has an effect on the amount of calories you naturally burn because muscle tissue requires more energy than fat.

The more muscle you have and the less fat present in your body, the faster your metabolism operates.[6]

---

[5] https://www.ncbi.nlm.nih.gov/pubmed/18448177; https://www.ncbi.nlm.nih.gov/pubmed/19640952

[6] https://www.ncbi.nlm.nih.gov/pmc/articles/PMC4258944/

It's been said a few times already fat loss is achieved by forcing the body to burn fat as a result of a caloric deficit. We've also said that the body turns not only to fat, but to muscle when it has energy requirements it needs to fulfill.

Although the intake of a certain amount of carbohydrates can curb the use of muscle tissue as an energy source, it is really important to continue to fill the body with protein to maintain the muscle in your body. Eating protein ensures that you continue to burn fat while keeping your muscle.

Another benefit of heavier protein consumption is that your body takes longer to digest, which requires the use of more energy in the process, and protein keeps you full for long periods of time.

When an individual eats a lot of protein with few carbohydrates, the metabolism changes and is placed into a state of **Ketosis**, which is another word to describe the process of burning fat rather than carbohydrates as an energy source.

Some great sources of protein include greek yogurt, eggs, steak, chicken, turkey, fish, beans, lentils, and quinoa.

In Summary:

1. The more protein you fill your muscles through protein consumption, the faster your metabolism works.
2. Protein helps ensure you burn fat while retaining muscle.
3. Protein keeps you full for longer periods of time, and keeps the digestive process active.

Fats

Your body requires you to eat fat in order to burn fat. It is indispensable to eat some forms of healthy fats. **Essential fats** keep your skin and hair healthy, and are integral to hormone production.

"Good fats" are titled "essential" because the body can't produce them on its own, or work properly without them. They're also important for brain development, and controlling inflammation in the body.

"Bad fats" or "saturated/trans fats" have no true nutritional value and, in fact, harm the basic processes they're meant to help facilitate.

Healthy fat consumption can come from vegetable oils, all sorts of nuts, avocados, eggs, chia seeds, fatty fish, coconuts (in addition to coconut oil), peanut butter, seeds, greek yogurt, and even dark chocolate.

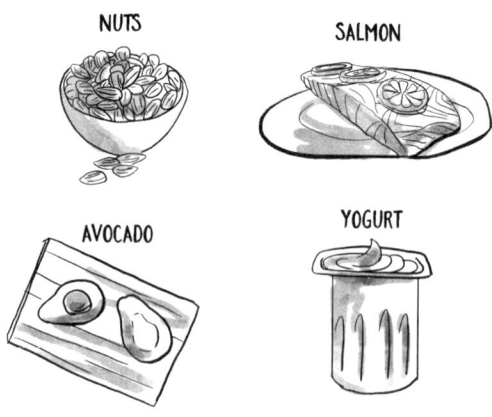

Different Ways To Track Your Nutrition

There are many ways to go about achieving your nutrition goals and you should be constantly experimenting to see which one is **the most realistic long-term option for you.**

 Using A More Intuitive Approach

There are many ways to take on a more intuitive eating approach and still achieve a healthy, happy body. Some of these are:

- Only eating foods when you're actually hungry
- Only eating foods that make you feel light and energetic afterwards
- Eating lots of vegetables and lean protein

Upsides	Downsides
- No need to do extra work like counting calories - Listening to your body generally provides useful guidance - Less of a mental strain on your eating decisions, provides a more flexible / relaxed process	- Easy to misread your body's signals and overeat or eat poorly - Without as much hard data, it's more difficult to adjust your results if you are not moving towards your long-term goal - Provides a gray area that is easy to make excuses and get past mentally

Using a More Meticulous, Scientific Approach

On the other end of the equation, you can use a more proven, science-based approach, which has its own benefits and flaws. This approach entails:

- Estimating how many calories you burn on a daily basis
- Tracking your daily caloric and macronutrient (macro) intake to either gain muscle or lose fat

Upsides	*Downsides*
- Guarantees optimal results when followed properly - Provides clear, black-or-white boundaries for you to follow - Forces you to really learn what foods are good for you by reading nutrition labels - Tracking your food promotes mindfulness and self-accountability	- Has a larger learning curve - A lot of extra work in reading nutrition labels and tracking everything - Difficult to estimate calories for some foods - Can be done excessively, leading to a harmful mental obsession

There are different degrees to which you can take this approach as well. On one end, you could start Googling nutrition facts for the foods you eat, get a rough idea of how many calories they are, and do mental math to quickly estimate everything. You have to be okay with some layers of inaccuracy in order to do this and trust yourself to adjust over time if your results aren't meeting your goals.

On the other hand, you could use a scale to measure exactly how much of each food you are eating in order to guarantee proper tracking. This approach can often be excessive and requires lots of extra work.

To be honest, there is so much gray area when it comes to food and nutrition tracking. It really comes down to personal preference and experimentation to find what works for you.

Keep in mind you can **incorporate elements of both approaches,** such as only counting calories, eyeballing your macronutrients, and always listening to your body's guidance.

You should also be **open to altering your plan over time.** For example, you could start with a more meticulous approach of counting calories + macronutrients, then once you reach your goal, switch to a more intuitive approach to maintain your weight, body fat, and muscle at your desired levels.

In the following section, we'll break down all the details of the latter approach so you can have all the information you need to get started with it.

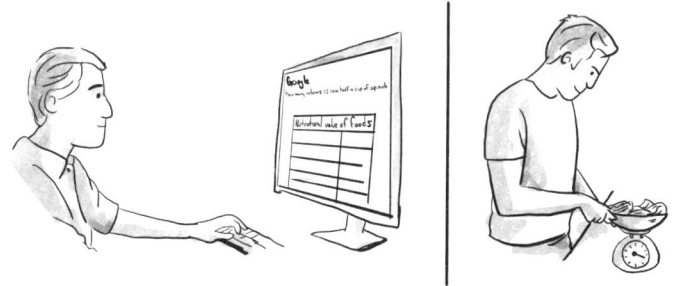

An Easy Start to Calorie Counting

Many people are afraid of counting calories as it is commonly thought of to be a very difficult option. Although there is a bit of a learning curve, it is a skill you can build for life, with minimal time investment.

Once you understand the basics of calorie / macronutrient counting, you'll be able to **near-guarantee your nutrition results** and spend **no more than 5 minutes a day** doing so.

If this is something that interests you and you'd like to try it out for 1-2 days, here are some great starting points:

1. Spend 15 minutes Googling "calories in [food name]", e.g. "calories in an apple". Do this for all the foods you most commonly eat so you have a great baseline going forward.

2. Download a calorie counting app - this lets you type in what food you ate, and although not completely accurate, will often help give you measurements on a food and an idea of its macronutrient breakdown, to boot. We recommend MyFitnessPal or Lifesum (no affiliation to either).

3. For starters, don't worry about macronutrient tracking, just stick to calories and see what it's like for a few days.

The benefit of starting with the more difficult step of tracking closely and seeing the results on the body are huge. You'll know the exact data (assuming you recorded it properly) that led to specific results. This will help you find out things like how your body reacts to a certain caloric input and macronutrient levels and lets you adjust over time if need be.

Calculating Your Daily Caloric Burn

Now that we know how to categorize the foods we eat, exactly how those foods affect our body, and how we can manipulate our body to force it to burn fat, we can get into the fun part… numbers!

The Basal Metabolic Rate

The first step in planning the best diet for you to burn the most fat starts with determining the number of calories you currently burn naturally, based on your activity levels.

Then, we can see what your diet needs to look like for you to obtain a caloric deficit. Ultimately, we'll calculate your ideal macronutrient ratio.

Each of us has a **Basal** (or Basic) **Metabolic Rate** – that is, we have a certain number of calories we'd each burn naturally on a daily basis, even if we were to lie in bed all day long. This is because our bodies expend a certain amount of energy by simply being alive and undergoing the physiological processes that need to occur for us to remain alive and function properly (respiration, digestion, etc.).

With regards to *achieving weight loss* **and** *preventing weight gain*, the higher your BMR is, the better it is.

The more calories your body naturally burns on its own without physical stimulation, the easier it will be for you to lose weight from a caloric standpoint.

As we grow older, our BMR starts to slow down (like every other bodily process).

But we can maintain and even speed our BMR up by regularly engaging in cardiovascular exercise. Jogging, running, biking, weight-lifting… any exercise that gets your heart rate up will increase the speed at which your body naturally burns calories – provided you do the activity regularly.

Calculating Your Basal Metabolic Rate:

1. 10 * _____ = _____   (Note: 1kg = 2.2lbs)
   (Weight in kg)

2. 6.25 * _____ = _____   (Note: 1 inch = 2.54cm)
   (Height in cm)

3. 5 * _____ = _____
   (Age in years)

4. _____ + _____ = _____
   (Step 1 Answer) (Step 2 Answer)

5. _____ - _____ = _____
   (Step 4 Answer) (Step 3 Answer)

6. For Females: _____ - 161 = _____
   (Step 5 Answer)   (Your BMR!)

6. For Males: _____ + 5 = _____
   (Step 5 Answer)   (Your BMR!)

If you need help with this, you can use an online BMR calculator for help. The link below provides one of the more accurate ones:
https://habitnest.link/bmrcalculator

Applying the Harris Benedict Formula

Having your BMR is great, but it's missing a key component: your daily activity through exercise. We can estimate this value using the Harris Benedict Formula.

To get to the actual number of calories you should be eating daily to maintain your current weight, you need to multiply your BMR by the appropriate factor in the Harris Benedict multiplier to get your overall energy expenditure in kilocalories a day.

See which choice reflects your lifestyle best:

Sedentary: BMR * 1.2
Little to no exercise

Mild Activity Level
BMR * 1.3 to 1.375 (Range)

Intensive exercise for at least 20 minutes, 1 to 3 times per week. This may include such things as bicycling, jogging, basketball, swimming, skating, etc. If you do not exercise regularly, but you maintain a busy **lifestyle** *that requires you to walk frequently for long periods, you meet the requirements of this level.*

Moderate Activity Level:
BMR * 1.5 to 1.55 (range)

Intensive exercise for at least 30 to 60 minutes, 3 to 4 times per week. Any of the activities listed above will qualify.

Heavy or Labor-Intensive Activity Level: BMR * 1.7

Intensive exercise for 60 minutes or greater, 5 to 7 days per week (see sample activities above). Labor-intensive occupations also qualify for this level.

Extreme Activity Level: BMR * 1.9

Exceedingly active and/or very demanding activities. Examples include: athlete with an almost unstoppable training schedule, with multiple training sessions throughout the day or a very demanding job, such as shoveling coal.

Calculating Your Total Daily Caloric Burn:

_____ * _____ = _____
(Your BMR)   (Harris Benedict   (Total Daily
               Multiplier)   Caloric Burn!)

The number you get above is the ceiling of calories you can eat daily without gaining weight.

This is of course assuming that you consistently maintain your current physical activity level. Getting to this number is an extremely important part of the fat-loss process. If you don't know how many calories you naturally burn a day, how can you ever figure out how many calories you'll need to eat to lose weight?

To be at a **caloric deficit** would mean that you either eat less than the number of calories you get out of the formula, or you exercise more.

Either way, you need to burn more than the number that results.

We will calculate how many calories you should eat daily to hit your goals in the next section.

In Summary:

1. Each one of us has a certain amount of calories we burn every single day by simply being alive.
2. You determine that number by determining your Basal Metabolic Rate and multiplying that number by the correct Harris Benedict Multiplier.
3. To enter into a caloric deficit, you would need to consume less (or burn more) than the number that results from the Harris Benedict Equation.

Calculating Your New Daily Caloric Intake

Now that we have total daily calories burned, we can see how many total calories you should eat daily to attain your goal.

If your **end goal is to get lean and gain muscle:**

We recommend getting to a low body fat % first (8-15% for men, 12-20% for women) via a caloric deficit (see below) before going into a slight caloric surplus (150-300 calories).

If your **end goal is to lose fat and maintain muscle**, you should enter a caloric deficit. How big of a deficit will depend on how quickly you want to see results and how realistic it is for you to consistently stick to those eating goals.

For a light caloric surplus (recommended for a more relaxed process)
- 10% daily caloric deficit
- Slower results
- Easiest option to maintain in the long-term
- Requires low amount of resistance training to minimize lost muscle tissue

For a medium caloric deficit (recommended for a time-sensitive goal)
- 20% daily caloric deficit
- Moderately fast results
- Medium difficulty to maintain
- Requires moderate amount of resistance training to minimize lost muscle tissue

For a high caloric deficit (not recommended)
- 30% daily caloric deficit
- Very fast results
- Requires high amount of resistance training to minimize lost muscle tissue
- Most difficult option, highest chance for binge-eating and hunger cravings. Requires very high willpower and discipline.

Any caloric deficit higher than 30% is **absolutely not recommended,** and we have a personal vendetta against such eating patterns… Mainly because of how much Mikey (one of the co-authors of this book) tried them, yo-yo dieted, lost a ton of muscle in the process, heavily slowed down his metabolism, and ended up with even higher body fat months later. For the sake of your ability to enjoy food in the long-term, stick to a 10-20% caloric deficit!

Calculating Your New Daily Caloric Intake

_____ * _____ = _____
(Total Daily   (10% to 30%)   (Caloric Deficit)
Caloric Burn)

_____ - _____ = _____
(Total Daily   (Caloric Deficit) (Your New Daily
Caloric Burn)   Caloric Intake!)

To prioritize building muscle, add 150-300 calories to your Total Daily Caloric Burn in place of the above calculations.

Now that we have the total calorie intake for each day, let's figure out what the macronutrient breakdown for it will be!

Calculating Your Macronutrient Ratio: How Much to Eat from Each Category of Food

Now that you have a good estimate of the amount of calories you need to be eating (or eating and burning) per day, you can properly determine the proper macronutrient ratio.

Macronutrient #1: Protein

Protein is a good place to start because of the importance of protein in your diet. Figuring out exactly how much protein you need to be eating per day to fall into the right balance in terms of forcing your body to burn fat while preserving muscle really depends on what your goals are for your body.

But generally speaking, 0.8 to 1 gram of protein **per lean mass of body weight** is usually more than enough for most people.[7] **Lean body mass** refers to the amount of weight you carry on your body that isn't fat.

In order to accurately calculate your lean body mass, we need to figure out your body fat %. There are a few different methods of doing this.

1. Get a measuring tape & use this link: https://habitnest.link/mtbf
2. Purchase an Accu-Measure self-measuring caliper from Amazon (Should be roughly $10. Note: We have no

---

[7] https://www.healthline.com/nutrition/how-much-protein-per-day#muscles-and-strength

affiliation with them, we simply think they have a great product.)

3. Alternatively, you can see if your local gym can do it for you for free.

4. Eyeball it using this picture: https://habitnest.link/bfpics

Once you have your body fat %, you can calculate your lean body mass by doing the following calculation:

Calculating Your Lean Body Mass[8]

1. _____ * _____ = _____
   (Current Weight)   (Body Fat %)   (Fat Weight)

2. _____ - _____ = _____
   (Current Weight)   (Fat Weight)   (Your Lean Body Mass!)

If you're trying to pack on muscle, the goal is to hit 1-1.5 grams of protein per pound of lean body mass.

By the same token, if muscle growth isn't quite as important to you, then 0.8 grams of protein per pound of lean body mass should be more than enough.

Remember though, even if you're not trying to gain any sort of muscular build, it is imperative to consume an adequate amount of protein to prevent existing muscle tissue from deteriorating. Based on your goals, you should choose which protein multiplier to use (somewhere between 0.8 and 1.5).

---

[8] https://en.wikipedia.org/wiki/Lean_body_mass

Calculating Your Daily Protein Intake

1. _____ * _____ = _____
    (Lean Body Mass) (0.8 to 1.5) (Your Daily
    　　　　　　　　　　　　　　　　　Protein Intake in g)

2. 4 * _____ = _____
    　　(Step 1 Answer) (Your Daily Protein
    　　　　　　　　　　　Intake in calories)

The above gives you your protein intake in grams per day. You can multiply this by 4 to get the total calories from protein that you should be eating each day.

Protein is by far the most important macronutrient to track, mainly because of how difficult it is to get the proper protein intake each day.

If you think tracking daily macronutrient intake is a bit overwhelming, you can just focus on getting the right protein intake and let carbohydrates and fats fall into place naturally - they will usually do so by themselves.

Fats

As we discussed, fats are really important to a number of our bodily processes. That being said, a good range of fats in one's diet is from 20-25% of the total calorie intake.[9] [10]

---

[9] https://www.ncbi.nlm.nih.gov/pmc/articles/PMC2763382/

[10] https://my.clevelandclinic.org/health/articles/11208-fat-what-you-need-to-know

If you enjoy more foods with fats in your diet, you can go towards the upper range of this. Otherwise, 20% will work well.

Calculating Your Daily Fat Intake

1. _____ * _____ = _____
   (Total Daily Caloric Intake)   (0.2 to 0.25)   (Your Daily Fat Intake in Calories)

2. _____ / 9 = _____
   (Step 1 Answer)   (Your Daily Fat Intake in Grams)

Carbohydrates

Now that we've **properly** come to the correct values for protein and fat consumption, figuring out the number of carbs that should be eaten to stay at a caloric deficit with a well-rounded diet is simple.

You can simply take your Total Daily Caloric Intake and subtract your Daily Fat Intake of Fat & Protein (in calories) from it.

Calculating Your Daily Carbohydrate Intake

1. _____ + _____ = _____
   (Daily Fat Intake in Calories)   (Daily Protein Intake in Calories)

2. _____ - _____ = _____
   (Your Daily Caloric Intake)   (Step 1 Answer)   (Your Daily Carb Intake in calories)

3. _____ / 4 = _____
   (Step 2 Answer)   (Your Daily Carb Intake in g)

You should now have all the calculations for exactly how much you should be eating on a daily basis, and of what nutrients! Of course it's difficult to hit these numbers exactly on a daily basis, but you should now have a fantastic guidance point.

To summarize, fill in the following values:

<u>**My Ideal Macronutrient Intake**</u>

Daily Caloric Intake: _____
(calories)

Daily Protein Intake: _____ _____
(grams) (calories)

Daily Fat Intake: _____ _____
(grams) (calories)

Daily Carb Intake: _____ _____
(grams) (calories)

As time goes on, feel free to experiment with different ratios of macronutrients to find your personal best long-term balance. These recommendations are of course just a starting point.

Note: If you're having trouble calculating your macronutrient ratio, BMR, or any other number, email support@habitnest.com. We'll guide you through it, or do it for you :).

Reading Nutrition Labels Like a Pro

Once you properly know your way around a nutrition label, you can scan them in seconds and know exactly how well a food fits within your dieting goals.

There are two parts to reading a nutrition label. The first is reading through the ingredients to see what's actually inside. Let's use an ice-cream alternative, Halo Top™[11], as an example (no affiliation).

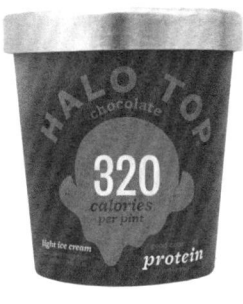

INGREDIENTS:

Skim milk, eggs, erythritol, cream, organic cane sugar, milk protein concentrate, high fat cocoa, vegetable glycerin, prebiotic fiber, sea salt, organic carob gum, organic guar gum, organic stevia leaf extract.

You can check the ingredients to see if there are processed, unhealthy, or other types of foods you want to avoid inside.

The ingredients are listed by quantity used, so we know that skim milk and eggs are the top two ingredients here. Note that Halo Top™ also has erythritol and stevia leaf extract which are zero-calorie sweeteners. If you really want to get

---

[11] https://halotop.com/flavors

Nutrition Facts

Serving Size 1/2 Cup (64g)
Servings Per Container 4

Amount Per Serving

Calories 80   Calories from Fat 25

% Daily Values*

Total Fat 2.5g	4%
Saturated Fat 1.5g	8%
Trans Fat 0g	
Cholesterol 45mg	15%
Sodium 110mg	5%
Total Carbohydrate 13g	4%
Dietary Fiber 2g	8%
Sugars 6g	
Sugar Alcohol 5g	
Protein 5g	10%
Vitamin A 2%	Vitamin C 0%
Calcium 10%	Iron 2%

*Percent Daily Values are based on a 2,000 calorie diet.

knowledgeable about what you're consuming, a Google search of the unfamiliar ingredient names can help shed some light. If you want to properly count calories and macronutrients, the nutrition label is typically where you'll spend most of your time.

The first step is to always **multiply** the **Servings Per Container** by the **calories, fat, carbs, and protein**. So:

4 (servings per container) * 80 (calories per serving) = 320 calories per container. Repeat this for the macronutrients and you get 10g of fat, 52g of carbs, and 20g of protein.

So if you ate the entire Halo Top™ container, you'd add to your daily intake:
320 calories, 10g of fat, 52g of carbs, and 20g of protein.

Since protein is often the most difficult macronutrient to get the most of, paying a bit more attention to what ratio of calories comes from protein is important.

Per serving, 5g of protein = 20 calories. 20 calories out of 80 total = 25% protein, making Halo Top™ a good source of protein (but a bad source of other important micronutrients and vitamins).

Calculating Your Ideal Water Intake

As a general rule of thumb, we can calculate your ideal water intake by multiplying your body weight by 0.67 and adding 0.4 ounces for each minute that you exercise each day.

This will give you your ideal water intake in ounces, which you can also convert to mL (whichever is easiest for you to track)

1. _____ * 0.67 = _____
   (Your Weight in Pounds)

2. 0.4 * _____ = _____
   (Average Minutes of Daily Exercise)

3. _____ + _____ = _____
   (Step 1 Answer) (Step 2 Answer) (Daily Water Intake in fl oz)

   1 fl oz = 29.6mL
   1 fl oz = 0.125 cups

*Note, this is a ROUGH estimate. How much water we each personally need is more dependent on differences within our lifestyle, daily circumstances, current weight, and body fat %. That being said, this serves as a good baseline and is likely just around what is optimal for you.

Ultimately, use your judgement here and consult your doctor and/or a nutritionist to verify what's best for you.

Now that we've covered all the bases of nutrition, let's learn a bit more about habits and how you'll be using the journal!

Effective Eating Styles to Try

There are many styles of diets that can help give you some structure on what you want to eat daily. We'll go over some of them and their pros/cons below. It's worth mentioning that **these are not all-or-nothing** styles of eating. You can definitely try some for a while, then take aspects that you enjoy and apply them to your long-term eating patterns without strictly following only that diet.

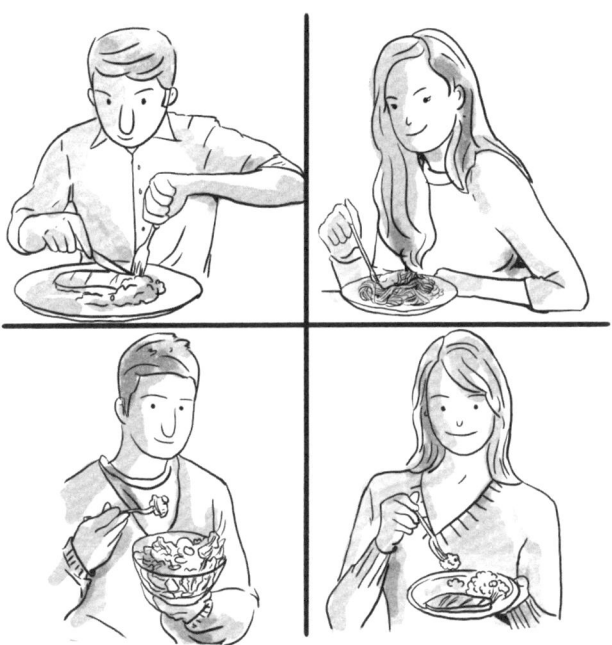

If It Fits Your Macros

The "IIFYM" eating style is essentially what we recommended earlier in this section, where you eat any foods you'd like as long as they lead to staying within the macronutrient range that will lead to your goals.

Upsides

- The most flexibility when it comes to what foods you can eat
- Easier to stick to during special events and occasions
- Provides little margin of error when followed properly
- Easy to adjust week-to-week to recalibrate towards your goals as you'll have lots of daily data points to work with

Downsides

- The largest learning curve of not just counting calories but also counting macronutrients
- Requires constant tracking of everything you eat
- Will never be 100% accurate
- The extra leniency can give too much leeway in eating, leading to breaking your daily limit

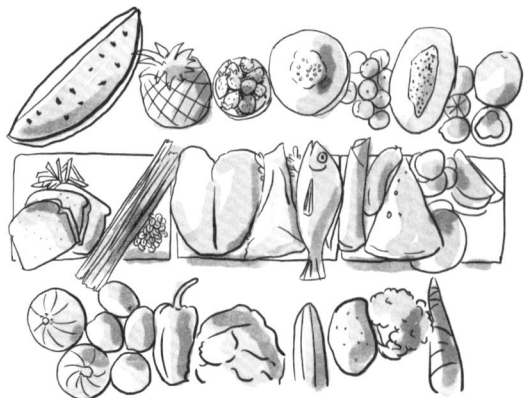

Paleo

Eating a paleo diet entails eating foods that are available in nature, just like our ancestors did in the early days of the human race. Advocates for paleo base their food choices on the idea that our bodies were not meant to handle the loads of processed foods that we tend to consume on a daily basis.

Upsides

- Simple guidelines to follow to stick to the diet
- Naturally leads to eating more lean protein and vegetables which can be healthy for many
- Indirectly promotes more meal-prepping as meals can be made rather simply with fewer ingredients
- Avoids many unhealthy food groups such as processed meats

Downsides

- Limited food choices as many food groups are prohibited
- Portion control becomes difficult since there are essentially no limits set, which could easily lead to overeating
- Difficult to follow for vegetarians or vegans, especially as beans/legumes are excluded
- Harder to maintain during special occasions

PALEO DIET

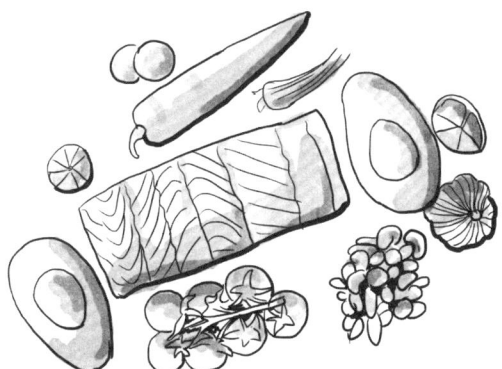

Keto

The keto diet predicates around drastically lowering carbohydrate intake and raising fat intake so your body enters a state of ketosis, which means it breaks down fat as its main energy source.

Upsides

- Has been consistently reported to increase mental clarity, energy, and help with autoimmune issues
- You'll primarily be eating delicious, calorie-dense, high-fat foods
- Drastically lowers sugar intake in the body

Downsides

- A very extreme diet with strict regulations and many banned food groups
- Has a longer ramp up time with reaching a state of ketosis
- Difficult to maintain long-term and at special occasions
- Optimal execution requires lots of self-experimentation, no clear answer

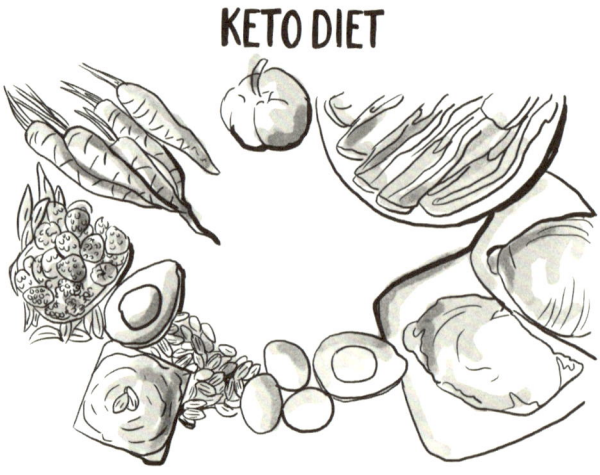

KETO DIET

Plant-Based

A plant-based diet involves... drumroll please... eating more foods that come from plants! You **do not have to be strictly vegetarian or vegan** to follow this, which provides a lot of great flexibility for people who generally love meat. There are some downsides with consistent meat consumption, such as increased ties to cancer from eating red meat (especially processed meats).[12] These can be minimized by introducing more of a plant-based meal system (e.g. only vegetables, beans, and eggs at lunch, no chicken, fish, or meat until dinner).

Upsides	Downsides
- Eating lots of vegetables for most meals is very healthy for you - Food is often cheaper if you are not including a meat option - Likely to have increase energy after meals due to the ease of digesting vegetables - Flexible: Can eat more plant-based meals in general without totally eliminating meat	- Meat products can be delicious and you will be eating less of them - May be difficult to get sufficient protein intake unless you turn to increased dairy or protein supplement intake - May not be as full after meals, leading you to fill up with more bread/carbs

PLANT-BASED DIET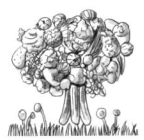

---

[12] https://www.who.int/features/qa/cancer-red-meat/en/

The Phases of Building a New Habit

The development of building a habit happens in stages. There's science behind all kinds of different theories about the stages that come along with altering habits, and here's what we found is the most accurate.

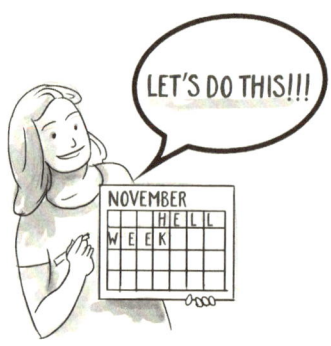

Days 1-7, **Hell Week.**

...*This part isn't fun.*

It isn't fun because you're beginning the process of rewiring a lifetime habit to be totally different. Expect HELL.

Days 8-21, Staying Consistent.

The good news is that after you've gotten through the first week, the process gets a lot easier. Hopefully, you've now figured out a few approaches that work. Your brain is beginning to understand the changes you're making and all the benefits that come with incorporating a cleaner diet into your daily routine.

During this period, a kick of inspiration can make all the difference. Developing habits takes time and just because you've surpassed the most difficult phase doesn't mean you're off the hook. In your journal, you'll be getting stories of successful people, how their diets have transformed their lives, along with daily challenges to keep you motivated and some more expert strategies along the way to keep the learning process going.

Days 21 - 66, Hardwiring - Retaining Interest in Your Personal Improvement.

Once you've passed phase 2, you know for a fact that YOU CAN DO THIS. It's amazing. All it takes is just about a month to add the habit, but that doesn't mean that phase 3 isn't crucial, because it is.

Your mind and your body will be used to saying no to garbage food that drain you of energy and life, you'll know the benefits of a wholesome nutrient-rich diet, but you still need to reach the point where it becomes the absolute norm.

During phase 3 you'll get really cool and interesting tools that you might find useful for staying consistent. We'll continue to provide you with stories of successful people for motivation, and we'll continue to sprinkle in affirmations along the way to keep your brain active in making your new healthy eating lifestyle a part of your DNA.

Days 66 and on, *Habit Mastery.*

At this point, you've built up the muscle memory for both the discipline healthy eating requires, along with the knowledge to create an effective, healthy eating plan. After building this skill once, it'll be that much easier to pick it back up at any future point in your life.

The Daily Content

Every single piece of content you're getting is a product of countless hours of sweat and research done by our team to ensure we're doing our best to:

- Light a fire in you to succeed in adding the habit.
- Provide you with the necessary knowledge and information to create a healthy diet that works for you.
- Make adding the habit fun and interesting.

Not only is every individual piece of content chosen amongst thousands of competing options, but the order of the content has been creatively designed to get you through the struggles associated with the different stages of adding habits.

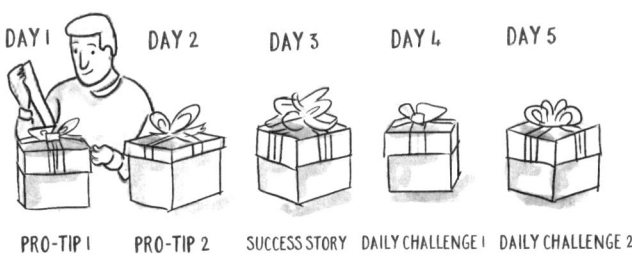

Here are the different types of content you can expect:

Pro-Tips

Pro-tips are the little golden nuggets of information you get to make implementing the habit on a day-to-day basis as simple and painless as possible. The point is to give you expert tips and hacks to get you going, and the variety and diversity of the different pro-tips will provide you with countless options for how to succeed in adding the habit.

Daily Challenges

The daily challenges you'll be receiving will be immensely important to your success in becoming a healthy eater.

Why?

They each help target a different area of discipline that will help you force yourself to do what's right - especially when you *don't feel like it.*

By strengthening this willpower-muscle inside you using small, very specific daily challenges, your self-discipline will grow more and more every single day. These daily challenges apply not just to **conquering your** diet but to all other aspects of your life - from curbing negative habits & distractions to building other healthy habits as well.

Clips & Podcasts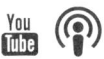

There's nothing as motivating as simultaneously seeing the passion in someone's eyes, hearing the truth in someone's voice, and feeling the intensity of their struggle. Connecting with people who have walked in your shoes and crossed over to the light of healthier eating habits will give you clear reference points that you can succeed at this just as others (amidst their own struggles) succeeded before you. Watching or listening to inspirational and informational content will serve as the informative reminder you need to get started and push through your normal, expected struggles until you've mastered this.

Success Stories

The reason we want to alter our habits is that we have an image of how much more incredibly wonderful our lives can be; how much better WE can be. When we hear stories about successful people who live their lives in accordance with the ways we want to change, it is motivating, inspiring, and gives us a high standard to live up to.

Successful people (whether physically, financially, emotionally, or spiritually) exhibit the same daily patterns… one of which is maximizing energy levels through healthy eating.

Getting bits and pieces of information about existing success stories will get you going on those days you don't feel you have it in you; those days where you just don't remember what you're aiming for anymore.

By having a successful icon's eating patterns dissected, you can also get ideas for how to improve your own diet.

We all need motivation, and understanding what it is that creates success for others will not only motivate you, but it will be a constant reminder of what it takes to be great.

Affirmations

Affirmations and visualization are highly effective tools used by some of the most successful people to have ever lived. From athletes to actors to CEOs, affirmations are used to help channel positive energy towards goals and create an inevitable connection between your present-self and the end goal you have in mind.

What affirmations really do:

- Subconsciously tap into your creativity muscle to begin generating creative ways of reaching your goals.

- Subconsciously program your brain to associate yourself with the end goal you have in mind, and prepares you to mentally sort out the steps necessary to get from where you are right now to your end goals.

- Attract you to your goal by the simple act of envisioning yourself where you want to ultimately be.

- Motivate you in the sense that it literally causes your brain to believe that you have within you the power, ability and capability to get exactly where you want in life.

So what does it mean to use affirmations?

Using affirmations is the act of repeating to yourself that you already are the person you want to be.

Envisioning that you can achieve your life goals, and you can be exactly the person you ideally envision yourself to be.

It is the repeating of idealistic situations you would like to see yourself in, except you say them in the present-tense, as if they were true now.

While repeating these affirmations, you visualize yourself as this ideal person, in the ideal situation you want to see yourself in, which trains your brain to believe it is possible.

The "How"

Perfectionists, Tread Lightly.
The Importance of Not Getting Caught up with Immediate Success

Sometimes there's a problem with shooting for perfection from the very start.

Shooting for perfection before you get through one day on a healthy diet can prevent you from ever taking one step in the direction of your goal.

So often you see people getting caught up in finding the best way to start working out, the best diet to lose weight, the most up-to-date research on the amount of sleep you need to be getting to feel amazing throughout the day...but we'll let you in on a little secret.

There's one simple concept that shatters all the best research, tips and strategies you can look for (all of the things that you'll be getting through this journal).

Here it is... the best way to become a healthy eater for life and form a diet that you can follow through with consistently...

You start doing SOMETHING.

You start taking SOME actions towards your goal.

You make SOME effort.

Don't let the desire to reach perfection - the possibility of having your goal body in a complete and wholesome way, disallow you from making sure you're making better eating decisions today than you did yesterday.

Don't waste your energy fantasizing and searching.

The best way to determine YOUR ideal healthy eating regimen is by starting to make small changes.

It's up to you to try ONE suggestion, and move forward from that point. Because altering your habits is about investigating what does and doesn't work FOR YOU, not for anyone else.

You'll be getting all the information and motivation you need from us on a daily basis in the form of daily content.

You won't PERSONALLY think every piece of content is useful. You won't think every tip will be effective. You won't think every podcast is insightful. You won't think every affirmation is worthwhile.

But if you make an attempt to use every piece of content, you'll see results. Pinky promise. Disregard the utility you *expect* out of it before trying it — take action first.

Every little action you take propels a snowball effect that greatly impact other areas of your life.

If you push yourself to follow your healthy eating routine for even 3 days, you're gifting yourself a positive chain of effects that will improve your daily energy, mental clarity, confidence, willpower, and overall quality of life.

In turn, when you don't prioritize the importance of your diet, each of these things get sacrificed. Building a consistent healthy eating routine is one of the most powerful tools you have to help you become the best version of yourself as quickly as possible.

Success is all about taking small, consistent actions over time.

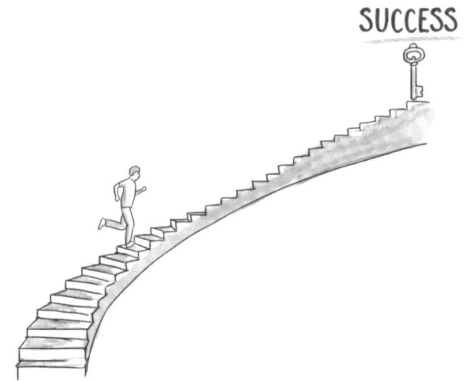

Important Notes on Mentality

Your brain has to change before your body can.

This journal is not meant to be a one-stop "diet" for weight loss. In fact, research conducted at UCLA that analyzed over 30 other long-term studies on dieting found that 33-66% of people who "diet" end up re-gaining more weight than they lost, regardless of the specifics of the diet. This is not an opinion. This is what the data shows.[13]

The true cost of following short-term weight loss solutions isn't merely wasted time, effort, and momentary suffering, it's all that plus further weight gain.

Our goal is to give you all the necessary tools and information for **changing your behavior** to lose weight and keep it off permanently. Small, sustainable and consistent change over time is the name of the game.

You have to rid yourself of the idea of perfection, and find a way to remove guilt and shame from this process - they will do nothing but destroy your intentions.

---

[13] http://newsroom.ucla.edu/releases/Dieting-Does-Not-Work-UCLA-Researchers-7832

Common Excuses to Overcome

At this point, you should know exactly *what* you need to do to get started. But sticking with that consistently is a whole different ball game.

Our brains tend to play lots of mental gymnastics that throw us off of our goals - especially with something so emotionally related as food. Some of these you should be ready for are:

1. Surpassing the mental barrier of **having to finish everything you take on your plate**

2. Surpassing the mental barrier that **having good food is rare and at special occasions you should eat as much as possible to take advantage of it.**

3. The mindset that if you ever go past your daily food goals, you've ruined your progress and **you may as well enjoy the full cheat meal and eat as many calories as possible.**

4. That your body is **different or special and conventional nutritional science doesn't apply to you.**

5. A lack of potential and belief that you can hit your goal.

6. Feeling **too pressured to hit your goal from a time perspective, then giving up.**

We've included these because these are all excuses we've found ourselves making. The quicker we were able to move past these false beliefs, the quicker we were able to build effective long-term changes.

You Are Perfect as You Are

In going through this process, it's really important to keep in mind that you are ALREADY perfect, and that increasing the quality of your daily life through food has nothing to do with your innate quality as a human being.

Eating or not eating certain foods and looking or not looking a certain way make you neither inferior nor superior to anyone else. Food keeps us alive and we live in a time where food is so accessible that we have the luxury to choose the foods we eat. Your food choices have nothing to do with you personally being 'good' or 'bad.' They are objectively related to your health, wellbeing, and weight loss.

Your end goal here isn't to be a certain weight, **it's to increase the quality of your emotional relationship with yourself**. You want to increase your energy levels, confidence, self-acceptance, and ultimately, love for yourself.

For that same reason, *forget about the number on the scale!* Looking good has nothing to do with an arbitrary number. The only time you need to step on a scale is every week or couple of weeks to see how any changes to your diet are affecting your weight - be objective about it.

Never forget that food is simply a vehicle for changing your mind and body. If you can get there regardless of food, you've won the true battle.

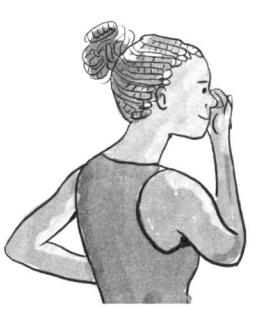 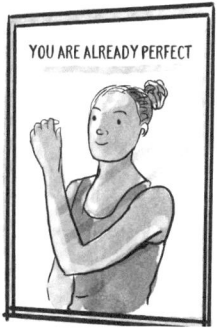

Sample Content Page

Day 32: **Pro-Tip**

Creative ways to satisfy your sweet tooth cravings.

Sweet food is DELICIOUS, and hunger cravings for them can sometimes feel so great to give in to, though they set us back very far on our goals. Here are some alternatives you can use to get over your sweet tooth cravings:

1. **Eat your berries!** Strawberries, blueberries, raspberries, blackberries, boysenberries, among others, are some of the best snacks to eat regularly and can help satisfy your sweet tooth. You can also try freezing your berries (or grapes)!

2. If you have an undying need to eat chocolate, **break off a piece of dark chocolate**, take it to another room, and let small pieces melt in your mouth (no chewing!) This can give you a few minutes of sweetness in your mouth for a lot less calories.

3. **Use See's Candies™ Lollypops** (no affiliation). These are available online at most retail outlets, have roughly ~90 calories, and can take 10-30 minutes to finish, satisfying your taste for having something sweet in your mouth for a very long time.

4. **Eat some coconut oil!** Although very high in calories (~100 per tbsp), it is incredibly effective at removing sweet tooth cravings.

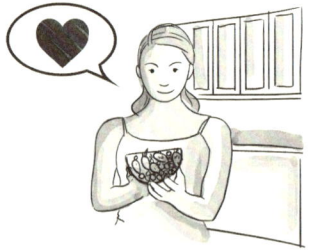

First we form habits; then they form us. Conquer your bad habits or they will conquer you." - Robert Gilbert

Sample Journal Page

DATE _____

⊕ TODAY'S NUTRITION GOAL

_____2,100 calories_____ ☑

◯ WATER DRINKING GOAL   🚶 EXERCISE GOAL

Two 500mL bottles ☑   _2 mile jog_ ☐

🍽 TODAY'S MEALS

📅 Planned	✓ Actual	Calories	Protein / Carbs / Fat
3 eggs w/ 2 rice cakes	3 eggs w/ 2 rice cakes	340	18g
Chicken + Broccoli + cauliflower	Burrito (tortilla, avocado, tomatoes, chicken)	800	1.5g
Salmon w/ asparagus	Salmon w/ asparagus	500	51g

🍎 SNACKS, DRINKS, & OTHER

30 almonds	210	9g
One snickerdoodle cookie	250	2.5g
TODAY'S TOTALS:	2,100	82g

🏃 POTENTIAL FOOD OBSTACLE(S) TO LOOK OUT FOR TOMORROW:

Resist the cookies at lunch!

⊕ ONE SMALL WAY I CAN IMPROVE MY NUTRITION TOMORROW IS:

If I bring a snack to work, I can eat that instead of sweets.

A Simple Idea

We hope that after reading the introductory pages, you're motivated and ready to tackle tomorrow morning with every ounce of energy you have.

We'll leave you to it with one simple idea.

Tomorrow, you will be exactly who you are **today**.

The rest of your life is a future projection of who you are today.

Only if you **change** today can tomorrow be **different**.

If you **don't change** today, the rest of your life is **pre-determined**.

Commit.

No matter what happens tomorrow…

*whether I am exhausted
or have the **worst** day of my life…*

*…whether I win the lottery
or have the **best** day of my life…*

I <u>will</u> eat healthier for the next week.

My word is like **gold**.

I will do whatever it takes
to make this happen.

_____

I will follow my eating goals (circle one):

      (**On Weekdays Only**)   (**Every Damn Day**)

_____   _____
Signature   Date

Progress Tracker (Optional)

| Progress Picture (Front) | Progress Picture (Side) |

How happy am I with myself (circle one)?

1   2   3   4   5

_____   _____
     Weight   Body Fat %

PHASE 1:
DAYS 1-7

Phase 1	Phase 2	Phase 3
Days 01-07	Days 08-21	Days 22-66+
Hell Week.	Staying Consistent.	Rewiring Your Brain.

Phase 1: Hell Week

When beginning a new habit, what's really important is getting to the point where you start to see the benefits you expect. It isn't going to be easy to start. You need to believe in yourself and take at least one concrete step in the direction of your goal every single day during this phase because it's really easy to lose hope right off the bat.

Make use of every tip, every affirmation, and all the motivation you're going to get to make it as easy as possible to take just one action towards your goal every day. Remember, we want to get to a point where we see benefits, and from that point on, the desire to re-acquire those benefits smoothens out the process.

Let's do this.

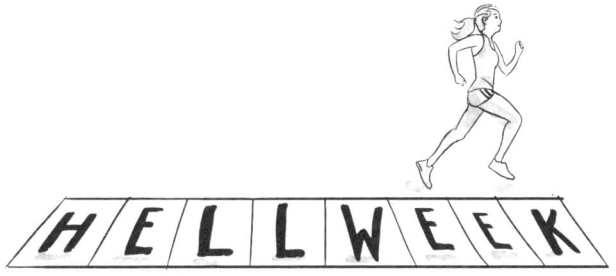

(Phase 1 Progress)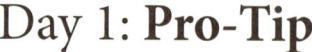

Day 1: **Pro-Tip**

Set your food goals the night before.

If you're deciding your meals right before you eat them, it's going to be very difficult to stick to any sort of healthy eating regimen. It's foolish to trust the hungriest version of you to make your food decisions when you want to create a habit of healthy eating and weight loss - we are completely unreliable on the spot. Deciding your meals the night before is the easiest way to avoid this fatal trap that causes most people to fail before they even start.

Each night, complete the following before going to bed:

1. Decide where you will eat each meal the next day, around what time, and what you will eat.
2. If you're counting calories and macros, check how well the nutrient breakdowns of the meals you plan to eat conform to your optimal daily intakes.

The point of this is to begin the learning process for how your body responds to different foods, and beginning to make a habit of taking action on your weight loss and health goals every day.

Superhero Option: Buy some Tupperware and make all of your meals for the next day before you go to bed - that way you know exactly what you're putting in your body!

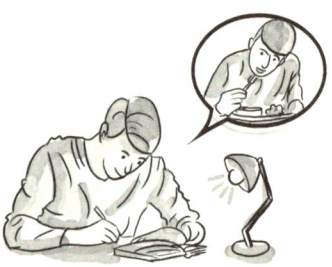

"To eat is a necessity, but to eat intelligently is an art." - La Rochefoucald

(Write your daily goal here, e.g. a calorie range, or a broader statement like "Only eat foods that make me feel great.")

🎯 TODAY'S NUTRITION GOAL

DATE _____

_____ ☐

💧 **WATER DRINKING GOAL** 🚶 **EXERCISE GOAL**

_____ ☐   _____ ☐

🍽 **TODAY'S MEALS** (Calorie & macronutrient tracking is 100% optional!)

📅 Planned	✓ Actual	Calories	Protein / Carbs / Fat

🍎 SNACKS, DRINKS, & OTHER

_____

_____

TODAY'S TOTALS: _____ _____

🏃 **POTENTIAL FOOD OBSTACLE(S) TO LOOK OUT FOR TOMORROW:**

_____

💡 **ONE SMALL WAY I CAN IMPROVE MY NUTRITION TOMORROW IS:**

_____

(Note: Anything not match up to your expectations for the journal? Email us at support@habitnest.com so we can make it right.)

Day 2: **Pro-Tip**

<u>Outsmart your hunger hormone.</u>

Even the most furiously motivated and focused dieters struggle with eating properly when hunger takes over. The hormone that controls how hungry we feel is called *ghrelin*. Ghrelin goes to work every 3-4 hours. When we skip meals and over-limit our carbohydrate intake, ghrelin secretion is heightened. We get *hangry* and have difficulty controlling how we eat.

This gets even more difficult when we sleep less than 7 hours as our ghrelin levels plummet, making us *ravenous*. Be VERY careful on days that you under sleep - your body will try to (ineffectively) restore your energy levels with food, instead of sleep or water.

We can control our body's ghrelin secretion by eating smaller, more balanced meals every 2-3 hours. Doing so keeps your metabolism working throughout the day, and controls your hunger levels so you're way less tempted to eat emotionally and out of control.

One easy way to implement eating every 2-3 hours is by splitting your lunch into two halves and eating them within a short time period.

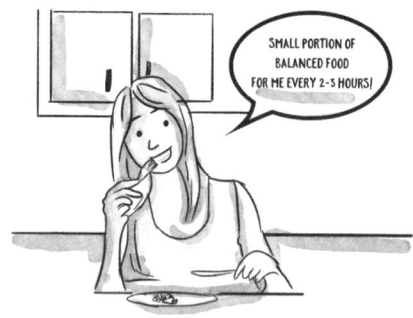

"All you need is love. But a little chocolate now and then doesn't hurt."
- Charles M. Schulz

TODAY'S NUTRITION GOAL   DATE

_____ ☐

WATER DRINKING GOAL   **EXERCISE GOAL**

_____ ☐   _____ ☐

(You can write your water drinking goal in any unit you prefer, e.g. mL, cups, oz, etc.)   **TODAY'S MEALS**

Planned	Actual	Calories	Protein / Carbs / Fat

SNACKS, DRINKS, & OTHER

_____

_____

(Food obstacle example: A social gathering where there will be a lot of temptation for unhealthy foods.)   TODAY'S TOTALS: _____

POTENTIAL FOOD OBSTACLE(S) TO LOOK OUT FOR TOMORROW:

_____

ONE SMALL WAY I CAN IMPROVE MY NUTRITION TOMORROW IS:

_____

(Life hack: If you use this journal's elastic band to hold it closed, the band doubles up as a pen holder. Slide your pen clip through it, allowing your pen to rest on top of the book!)

Day 3: **Daily Challenge** 🔥

Challenge: Pay attention to the mini-decisions you make today. Ask yourself, "If I made this choice EVERY DAY (for example, the decision to drink soda), would I be a lot closer to my goals, or a lot further?"

<u>Newsflash</u>: **Your choices are 100 times more important than you think.** Every choice you make today is building up a habit for the rest of your life. Our brains learn from what we do repeatedly - the decision to overeat is, in reality, 100x more powerful over time.

Taking one tiny action in a positive direction has the same effect. Not having that one soda or one candy bar, over time, is a BIG deal.

You can justify not sticking to your healthy eating regimen, but your mind and body grow accustomed to it. Your brain only knows **what you do**. When you start the day with intention, your brain rewires itself. *All mini-decisions build up to your habits.* **You** *are* **your mini-decisions.**

☐ I completed this daily challenge.

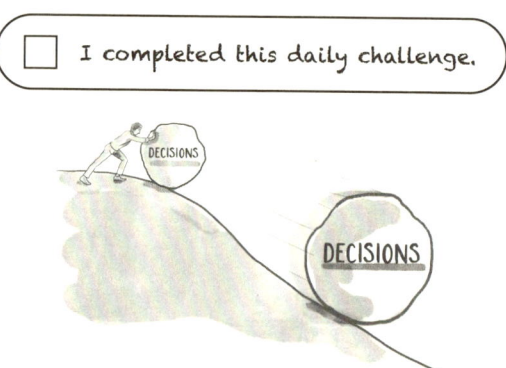

"Don't let the old you make your decisions. Today is the only day change exists. Change today, and your entire life will be altered. Don't change today, and tomorrow will be exactly like today, forever."
- Ari Banayan

⊕ **TODAY'S NUTRITION GOAL**   DATE

_____ ☐   _____

◊ **WATER DRINKING GOAL**   🚶 **EXERCISE GOAL**

_____ ☐   _____ ☐

(Although there's room for 5 meals a day below, fill in only as many as you actually eat in a day, which could be as low as 1-2 for people practicing intermittent fasting.)

📅 Planned	✓ Actual	Calories	Protein / Carbs / Fat

🍎 **SNACKS, DRINKS, & OTHER**

_____

_____

(You can include alcohol in the above snacks/drinks section as well.)   TODAY'S TOTALS: _____

🏃 **POTENTIAL FOOD OBSTACLE(S) TO LOOK OUT FOR TOMORROW:**

_____

💡 **ONE SMALL WAY I CAN IMPROVE MY NUTRITION TOMORROW IS:**

_____

(Improvement example: **remove** high calorie additions from my sandwich at **lunch**, like cheese or sauce.)

Day 4: **Pro-Tip**

Apply the three principles of nutrition to as many meals as you can.

Having fantastic nutrition breaks down to three main principles:

1. Eating foods that **taste great** to you
2. Eating foods that are nutritious and **good for you**
3. Eating foods that **make you feel great afterwards**

Right now, make a list of these foods for yourself. You should consistently be on the lookout for foods / meals that check off all these three boxes for you, and when you do, to start incorporating them more frequently into your meals.

This will ensure you will enjoy it, it will help you reach your goals, and will consistently help you feel great afterwards, both physically and emotionally. These foods definitely exist and are out there for everybody, but definitely vary from person to person.

You can also achieve this by using spices, lemon, or low-calorie sauces on otherwise bland-yet-healthy food.

Superhero option: for three days, ONLY eat foods that these apply to and nothing else. Then, see how you feel afterwards.

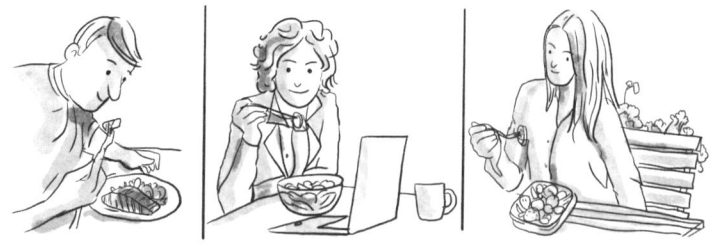

"Your diet is a bank account. Good food choices are good investments."
- Bethenny Frankel

TODAY'S NUTRITION GOAL

DATE

_____ ☐

WATER DRINKING GOAL **EXERCISE GOAL**

_____ ☐ _____ ☐

TODAY'S MEALS (Be specific about your exercise goal, e.g. 20 minute jog, hour of weightlifting, or morning walk.)

Planned	Actual	Calories	Protein / Carbs / Fat

SNACKS, DRINKS, & OTHER

_____

_____

TODAY'S TOTALS: _____ ____ ____ ____

POTENTIAL FOOD OBSTACLE(S) TO LOOK OUT FOR TOMORROW:

_____

ONE SMALL WAY I CAN IMPROVE MY NUTRITION TOMORROW IS:

_____

Day 5: **Pro-Tip**

Experiment with high-protein food alternatives.

Note: We have zero affiliation with any of the products below, we simply enjoy eating them and think they are great products.

Getting sufficient protein intake is usually the most difficult of all the three macronutrients. It is so easy to fill up on carbs and/or fat as they are usually the foods that are most readily available as snacks.

Finding high-protein foods that also taste great can be a magical find. We wanted to share some of our own personal favorites:

1. <u>Edamame Pasta</u>
   - Available at Costco or online, easy to make
   - Incredible protein ratio of ~45% (that's 15% more than an eggs!)
   - Con: Made of 100% soy which has reports of being unhealthy

2. <u>Cali'Flower Crusts</u>
   - Delicious pizza crust made of cauliflower + eggs + cheese
   - Available online, easy to make
   - Con: Expensive at ~$5 per crust

3. <u>Greek Yogurt</u>
   - Available at most local food stores
   - Incredible protein ratio of ~50%
   - We recommend mixing in berries, cinnamon, or PBFit powder

4. <u>Adding additional egg whites to an omelette</u>
   - Can make a breakfast meal a lot more dense and filling while adding almost straight protein

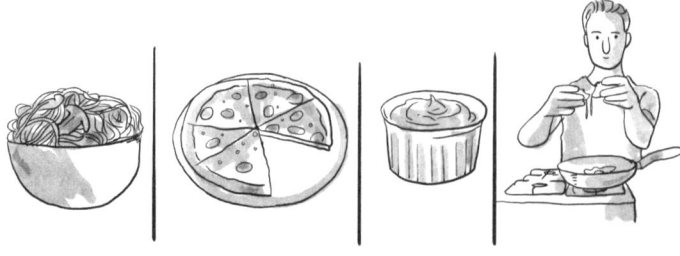

⊕ **TODAY'S NUTRITION GOAL**　　　DATE

_____ ☐

◌ **WATER DRINKING GOAL**　　　🚶 **EXERCISE GOAL**

_____ ☐　　　_____ ☐

🍴 **TODAY'S MEALS**

| 🗓 Planned | ⊘ Actual | Calories | Protein / Carbs / Fat |

🍎 SNACKS, DRINKS, & OTHER

_____

_____

TODAY'S TOTALS: _____

🏃 **POTENTIAL FOOD OBSTACLE(S) TO LOOK OUT FOR TOMORROW:**

_____

⏱ **ONE SMALL WAY I CAN IMPROVE MY NUTRITION TOMORROW IS:**

_____

Day 6: **Daily Challenge**

Challenge: Try intermittent fasting for a day.

Intermittent fasting can be a very powerful tool to help you achieve your nutrition goals. It consists of only eating within a 4-8 hour window each day.

Many people report not being hungry until noon or so, and that hunger during early morning hours was just something they had gotten used to before trying intermittent fasting.

In fact, in some countries in the world such as Greece, it is a cultural norm to not have breakfast at all and only start eating around lunchtime. Like in Greece, you can use coffee / tea in the morning hours to help get you through the morning until lunchtime.

One interesting tip is how different fields of thought conflict so much with each other. On one end of popular belief, people with incredible physiques say they got the best results eating frequent meals every 2-3 hours. On the other end, many people who follow intermittent fasting and eat 1-2 meals a day in a small window have great results too.

This is why nutrition is so individualized and it's so important to test different approaches to see what works best for your lifestyle.

☐ I completed this daily challenge.

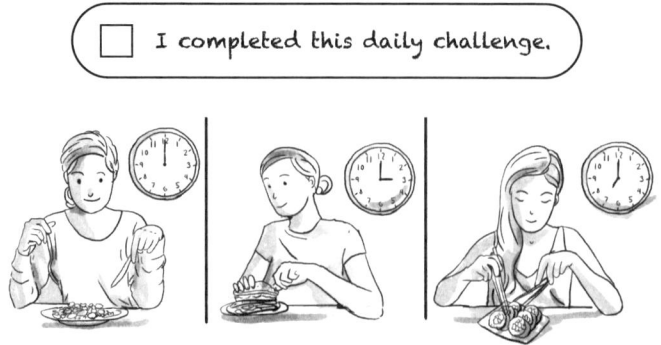

TODAY'S NUTRITION GOAL　　　　　　　　　DATE

_____ ☐

💧 **WATER DRINKING GOAL**　　🚶 **EXERCISE GOAL**

_____ ☐　_____ ☐

🍴 **TODAY'S MEALS**

📅 Planned　　　　✓ Actual　　　　Calories　Protein / Carbs / Fat

🍎 SNACKS, DRINKS, & OTHER

TODAY'S TOTALS: _____

🏃 **POTENTIAL FOOD OBSTACLE(S) TO LOOK OUT FOR TOMORROW:**

_____

🧭 **ONE SMALL WAY I CAN IMPROVE MY NUTRITION TOMORROW IS:**

_____

Phase 1 Complete!

Day 7: **Pro-Tip**
It's better in the trash than in your stomach.

You know how when we're young many of our parents tell us to finish our food so we don't 'waste' it? It's time to completely let go of that thought and realize that if you're not hungry, you should not be eating.

It is much more harmful to avoid 'wasting' food by eating it when you're not hungry than to throw it away, or to give to someone else who may actually be hungry. Even if you're on a really specific diet that requires you to eat every so often, avoid eating when you're not hungry at all costs (unless you're really trying to put on weight). Eating when we're not hungry distorts our understanding of what hunger is, which causes us to eat emotionally, and with our eyes, rather than listening to our stomach's direction.

To ingrain this as a habit, you can practice leaving the last bite of food on your plate each meal. This builds up your discipline with food, especially if it's with leaving a bite of food you normally crave.

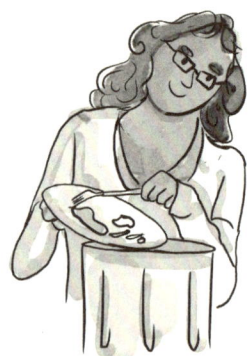

"Appetite has really become an artificial and abnormal thing, having taken the place of true hunger, which alone is natural. The one is a sign of bondage but the other, of freedom."
- Paul Brunton

TODAY'S NUTRITION GOAL   DATE

_____ ☐

💧 **WATER DRINKING GOAL**   🚶 **EXERCISE GOAL**

_____ ☐   _____ ☐

🍽 **TODAY'S MEALS**

📅 Planned   ✓ Actual   Calories   Protein / Carbs / Fat

🍎 SNACKS, DRINKS, & OTHER

TODAY'S TOTALS: _____ _____ _____

🏃 **POTENTIAL FOOD OBSTACLE(S) TO LOOK OUT FOR TOMORROW:**

⏱ **ONE SMALL WAY I CAN IMPROVE MY NUTRITION TOMORROW IS:**

~~PHASE 1:~~ CONQUERED.

Pssssttt... We like rewarding people (like you) who TAKE ACTION and actually use this journal. Email us now at secret+nutrition@habitnest.com for a secret gift ;)

Phase 1 Recap: Days 1-7

1. After looking at your tracking information for Phase 1, what have you personally learned about the relationship between your body and the food you eat?

_____
_____
_____
_____

2. Which strategies helped you stick to your regimen, and which strategies weren't useful at all?

_____
_____
_____
_____

3. What are some new strategies you want to experiment with?

_____
_____
_____
_____

4. If you continued this habit for another 2 weeks, how do you think you'll look and feel about yourself?

_____
_____
_____
_____

5. If you dropped this habit now, what do you stand to lose?

_____
_____
_____
_____

6. What are some irrational thoughts you have consistently about your body image? How can you improve the way you view yourself?

_____
_____
_____
_____
_____
_____
_____

PHASE 2:
DAYS 8-21

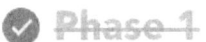 Phase 1 | **Phase 2** | Phase 3

Days 01-07
Hell Week.

Days 08-21
Staying Consistent.

Days 22-66+
Rewiring Your Brain.

Phase 2: Digging Deep - Staying Consistent

Congratulations, you've gotten through Phase 1 (Hell-Week). By this point you should have some idea of how to stick to your new healthy eating regimen, and how your body reacts to different types of food.

If you don't feel like you've made as much progress as you'd like, don't worry. One day at a time, one victory at a time is the name of the game.

Phase 2 is important because this is the point where we either feel like we've got it down OR, we feel hopeless that we'll never reach our goals.

Either way, ignore what your mind says. If you feel like you've reached your goal, don't trust the feeling because now you need to STAY consistent.

If you feel hopeless, you won't feel hopeless forever as long as you continue to believe in yourself and make a real effort every day.

Let's make big moves.

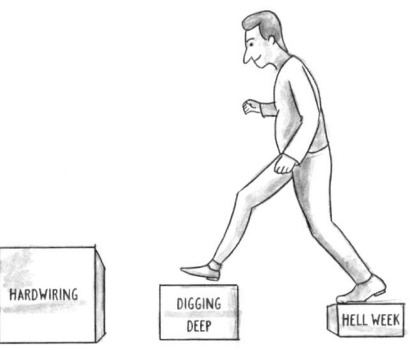

Commit.

*I KNOW this next phase
is going to be extremely hard.*

*I understand I may not
be perfect about it every day.*

*But I <u>will</u> put my heart, each day, into
conquering this life-changing goal.*

**If I miss a day,
I will pick back up.**

*Off days and missed days
will NEVER stop me.*

*In the long-run,
I will win.*

I will complete Phase 2 of this journal.

Signature   Date

Day 8: **Success Story**

Mikey Ahdoot, co-author of this journal.

To be honest, I'm a bit embarrassed typing this, though I am doing so in case my journey helps somebody else.

I LOVE FOOD. I slapped my cousin for taking a tortilla chip away from me when I was 3 and cried when my mom asked me to share my ravioli as a kid. I was the most overweight child in my elementary and middle school (and arguably the cutest). There has not been a day of my life that I haven't thought about my food choices since 9th grade, and there was so much I was insecure about with my body.

12 years later, I am still watching my food choices every day and I'm finally starting to make significant breakthroughs of consistently maintaining a healthy, happy body. The principles I use are many of the ones outlined in this journal. I'm up in muscle and down roughly 40 pounds of fat from my heaviest!

I write this to hopefully shift some person's mindset out there to:

1. Have a long-term vision of where you're going (e.g. **giving yourself years to achieve your goals**, instead of weeks or months), and
2. Practice **unconditional forgiveness of yourself** throughout the entire journey, through every binge-eaten meal, through every slip-up you have. Keep an insatiable drive to achieve your goal.

These are such huge, critical parts of this process. If you ever want to talk about anything in your journey, please email me directly at mikey@habitnest.com and I'll personally respond.

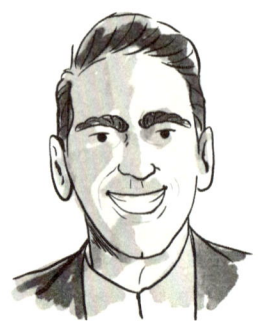

⊕ **TODAY'S NUTRITION GOAL** DATE

_____ ☐

◊ **WATER DRINKING GOAL**   ⚐ **EXERCISE GOAL**

_____ ☐   _____ ☐

🍴 **TODAY'S MEALS**

📅 Planned   ✓ Actual   Calories   Protein / Carbs / Fat

_____|_____   _____   _____

_____|_____   _____   _____

_____|_____   _____   _____

...........................|...........................   ....

...........................|...........................   ....

🍎 SNACKS, DRINKS, & OTHER

_____   _____   _____

_____   _____   _____

TODAY'S TOTALS: _____ _____ _____

✓ **BENEFITS I FELT TODAY (CIRCLE):**

Feel Happier   More Creative   Increased Willpower   Improved Focus   More Energized   Reduced Stress

Day 9: **Daily Challenge**

Challenge: Write down what factors have recently impeded you from successfully sticking to your eating goals.

Envision the most recent time you completely "failed" and gave into major cravings, or had some other negative experience with it.

Now breathe… everybody, and we mean ***everybody*** struggles with consistency. The truth is that imperfect days teach us the most about how to succeed.

Treat days you mess up as experiments. By consciously writing down what factors caused us to struggle, we can better prepare against them.

On days you aren't "perfect," try to answer these questions:

1. What was my thought process during the first decision I made that led me astray from my goal? What can I learn from this and apply moving forward?
2. In addition to the above, what are some additional "rules" I can set to prevent what caused this specific slip-up in the future?
3. What justification did I tell myself to make it okay to slip up?

These mental insights can really act as secret weapons on days we struggle. We will all miss our habits. Let's make those days just as valuable as perfect days by treating them as learning experiences.

☐ I completed this daily challenge.

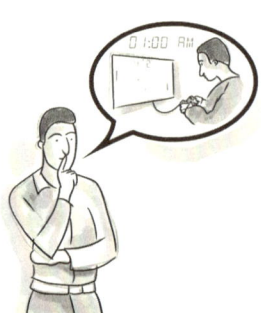

TODAY'S NUTRITION GOAL

DATE: _____

_____ ☐

WATER DRINKING GOAL   EXERCISE GOAL

_____ ☐   _____ ☐

TODAY'S MEALS

Planned	Actual	Calories	Protein / Carbs / Fat

SNACKS, DRINKS, & OTHER

_____

_____

TODAY'S TOTALS: _____

BENEFITS I FELT TODAY (CIRCLE):

Feel Happier | More Creative | Increased Willpower | Improved Focus | More Energized | Reduced Stress

Day 10: **Pro-Tip**

<u>Drink naturally flavored water.</u>

It is impossible to over-state the importance of water and understate the importance of getting rid of sugary drinks from your diet. If you can completely eliminate drinks with tons of sugar in them, you will almost immediately see the difference.

Water is an important part of all bodily functions and processes, it helps you feel full and keeps you feeling fresh and energized. The *Food & Nutrition Board* recommends drinking eight 8-ounce cups of water every day for optimal health for the average person.

Here are a couple of easy tricks to help you drink more water:

1. One AMAZING way to satisfy your sweet tooth and avoid drinks with sugar is to simply add completely natural fruits and vegetables to your water. Lemon, cucumbers, strawberries, blueberries, raspberries, pineapple… any natural fruit, no matter how weird it seems, will make a significant difference in the taste.

2. Buy a good refillable water bottle. Every time you want to get up to go to the bathroom, drink. Every time you get back to your seat from the bathroom, drink.

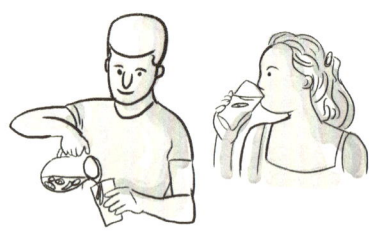

"There are two primary choices in life: to accept conditions as they exist, or accept the responsibility for changing them." - Dr. Denis Waitley

DATE _____

⊕ **TODAY'S NUTRITION GOAL**

_____ ☐

💧 **WATER DRINKING GOAL**   🚶 **EXERCISE GOAL**

_____ ☐   _____ ☐

🍽 **TODAY'S MEALS**

📅 Planned   ✓ Actual   Calories   Protein / Carbs / Fat

_____   _____ _____

_____   _____ _____

_____   _____ _____

....

....

🍎 SNACKS, DRINKS, & OTHER

_____

_____

TODAY'S TOTALS: _____ _____

✓ **BENEFITS I FELT TODAY (CIRCLE):**

Feel Happier   More Creative   Increased Willpower   Improved Focus   More Energized   Reduced Stress

Day 11: **Affirmations**

1. Find a quiet area where you can do this in private so you can do this at ease. If you can't find a private space, say these in your head while pretending you're screaming them from a mountaintop.

2. Think of a time where you felt absolutely powerful - **where you felt on top of the world**. Tap into every emotion you had at that moment and get yourself into that state right now. How were you feeling then - Powerful? Unstoppable? Strong? Incredible!? Get into it now!!!!

3. Now feel your intensity grow tenfold! Say this with deep passion:

My body is my sanctuary. I take care of my body by giving it foods that will make it operate at its highest potential and in turn my body feeds me with incredibly high levels of energy. Every day, I am stronger and healthier because I am willing to slow down and think about what I'm putting in my body. I nourish my body with what it deserves.

Repeat this **one more time**.

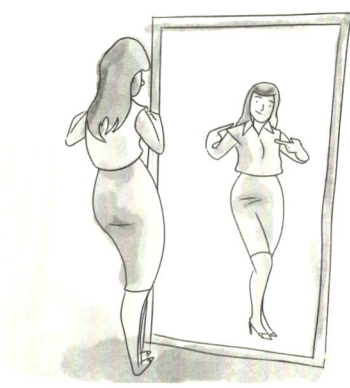

"The greatest wealth is Health."
-Unknown

TODAY'S NUTRITION GOAL

DATE

_____ ☐

WATER DRINKING GOAL   EXERCISE GOAL

_____ ☐   _____ ☐

TODAY'S MEALS

| Planned | Actual | Calories | Protein / Carbs / Fat |

_____
_____
_____
....
....

SNACKS, DRINKS, & OTHER

_____
_____

TODAY'S TOTALS: _____ _____ _____ _____

BENEFITS I FELT TODAY (CIRCLE):

Feel Happier · More Creative · Increased Willpower · Improved Focus · More Energized · Reduced Stress

Day 12: **Success Story**

Tony Robbins.

Tony Robbins has written multiple best-sellers and tens of thousands of people pay thousands of dollars to go to one of his many life-changing seminars every year. He continuously works on his own habits and his life's work is about helping people overcome their own limitations. One of the habits he heavily promotes is healthy eating.

"My number one health tip is to look after the delicate acid-alkaline balance in the body, which can be measured with a urine or saliva test. The easiest way to do that is to 'go green' by introducing lots of fresh green vegetables like spinach, broccoli, asparagus, cabbage and bok choy into your diet. The vast majority of organs, and especially your blood, have to be slightly alkaline for good health. This keeps oxygen flowing into the blood cells."

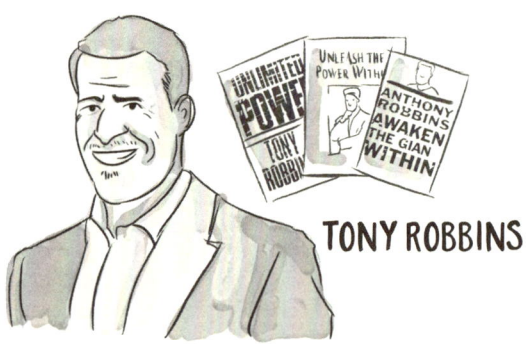

"Whenever you do a thing, act as if all the world were watching."
- Thomas Jefferson

TODAY'S NUTRITION GOAL

DATE: _____

_____ ☐

WATER DRINKING GOAL

_____ ☐

EXERCISE GOAL

_____ ☐

TODAY'S MEALS

Planned	Actual	Calories	Protein / Carbs / Fat

SNACKS, DRINKS, & OTHER

TODAY'S TOTALS: _____ _____

BENEFITS I FELT TODAY (CIRCLE):

Feel Happier   More Creative   Increased Willpower   Improved Focus   More Energized   Reduced Stress

Day 13: **Pro-Tip**

Eat a 'cheat' meal every few days instead of having full cheat days.

Most people have "cheat days" during which they eat whatever they want for a full day or weekend.

There are two problems with this. First, it makes it WAY harder to go back to eating healthy the next day. Second, a full day of garbage makes you feel like garbage for multiple days, and actually forces your body to crave the garbage that made it feel horrible in the first place.

If you can commit to just ONE completely unmonitored meal of your choice, one meal at a time every couple of days, you won't feel horrible for days on end, and it'll be easy to continue with your healthy eating regimen immediately after.

Another approach you can try is having two days a week where you maintain your weight instead of staying in a caloric deficit/surplus.

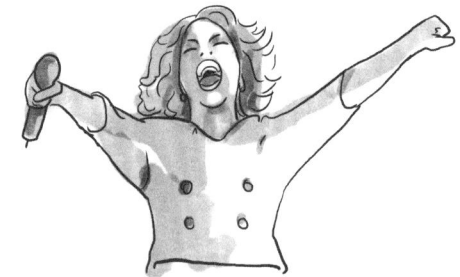

"Health is a relationship between you and your body" -Terri Guillemet

TODAY'S NUTRITION GOAL

DATE: _____

_____ ☐

WATER DRINKING GOAL

_____ ☐

EXERCISE GOAL

_____ ☐

TODAY'S MEALS

Planned	Actual	Calories	Protein / Carbs / Fat

SNACKS, DRINKS, & OTHER

_____

_____

TODAY'S TOTALS: _____

✓ BENEFITS I FELT TODAY (CIRCLE):

Feel Happier   More Creative   Increased Willpower   Improved Focus   More Energized   Reduced Stress

Day 14: **Favorite Resources** 🍴

Product: Fooducate (iPhone or android App)
Cost: Free

Note: we have no affiliation with Fooducate. We just love the app.

Fooducate is an awesome application that basically acts as a "food coach." Fooducate will scan barcodes on food items to break down its nutritional value and ingredients for you in real time. It also helps you stay on track by setting specific goals based on your body's current state of health.

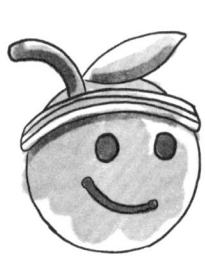 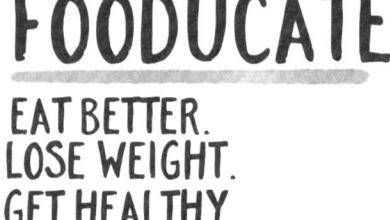

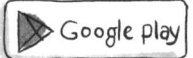 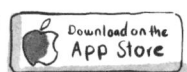

"To succeed you must first improve, to improve you must first practice, to practice you must first learn, to learn you must first fail."
- Wesley Woo

DATE _____

⊕ **TODAY'S NUTRITION GOAL**

_____ ☐

◊ **WATER DRINKING GOAL**   🚶 **EXERCISE GOAL**

_____ ☐   _____ ☐

🍽 **TODAY'S MEALS**

| 📅 Planned | ✓ Actual | Calories | Protein / Carbs / Fat |

🍎 SNACKS, DRINKS, & OTHER

TODAY'S TOTALS: _____

✓ **BENEFITS I FELT TODAY (CIRCLE):**

Feel Happier | More Creative | Increased Willpower | Improved Focus | More Energized | Reduced Stress

Progress Tracker (Optional)

```
┌─────────────────────┐   ┌─────────────────────┐
│                     │   │                     │
│                     │   │                     │
│   Progress Picture  │   │   Progress Picture  │
│       (Front)       │   │        (Side)       │
│                     │   │                     │
│                     │   │                     │
└─────────────────────┘   └─────────────────────┘
```

How happy am I with myself (circle one)?

1   2   3   4   5

_____   _____
Previous Weight   Previous Body Fat %

_____   _____
Weight   Body Fat %

Day 15: **Double Daily Challenge** 🔥

Challenge: Juice right after you get up.

Juicing in the morning is the EASIEST way to get a lot of your vegetable and fruit requirements out of the way early on. It also wakes you up and makes you feel really good before the day starts. You can literally make it any which way you want, but make sure there are tons of greens in there, along with fruit, for good taste.

Try this: Either set aside the fruits you want to use for your morning juice, or make the juice at night and stick it in the fridge.

Eat lower-calorie nighttime snacks.

The way we eat at night, especially right before bed, has a dramatic impact on our weight. We all know what it feels like to binge on ice cream, chips, candy or chocolate right before bed.

We challenge you to make a super-effort to avoid calorie-dense, carbohydrate rich foods before bed. Replace them with light, low-calorie vegetables and fruits. You'll quickly see that "zero" or close to "zero calorie foods" like celery, broccoli, grapefruit, lettuce, lime, lemon and cabbage, will actually help you lose weight. You'll wake up thinner and lighter. At the very least, try it tonight!

☐ I completed this daily challenge.

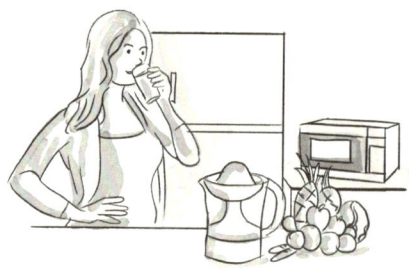

⊕ **TODAY'S NUTRITION GOAL**   DATE

_____ ☐

○ **WATER DRINKING GOAL**   🚶 **EXERCISE GOAL**

_____ ☐   _____ ☐

🍽 **TODAY'S MEALS**

📅 Planned   ✓ Actual   Calories   Protein / Carbs / Fat

_____|_____   _____ _____

_____|_____   _____ _____

_____|_____   _____ _____

.......................|.......................   ....

.......................|.......................   ....

🍎 SNACKS, DRINKS, & OTHER

_____

_____

TODAY'S TOTALS: _____ _____

✓ **BENEFITS I FELT TODAY (CIRCLE):**

Feel   More   Increased   Improved   More   Reduced
Happier   Creative   Willpower   Focus   Energized   Stress

Day 16: **Affirmations**

1. Find a quiet area where you can do this in private so you can do this at ease. If you can't find a private space, say these in your head while pretending you're screaming them from a mountaintop.

2. Think of a time where you felt absolutely powerful - **where you felt on top of the world**. Tap into every emotion you had at that moment and get yourself into that state right now. How were you feeling then - Powerful? Unstoppable? Strong? Incredible!? Get into it now!!!!

3. Now feel your intensity grow tenfold! Say this with deep passion:

I listen to my body when it tells me that it is satisfied. My taste buds are slowly changing every day and I no longer crave foods that don't nourish me. I choose health and wellness over the temporary mental satisfaction of sugar and fat. I feel amazing when I take care of my body. When I take care of my body, my body takes care of me.

Repeat this **one more time.**

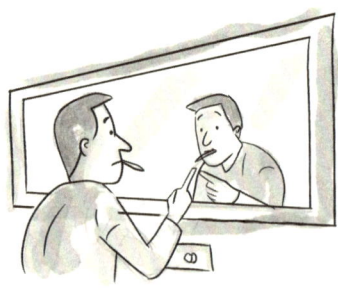

"Experience tells you what to do; confidence allows you to do it."
- Stan Smith

TODAY'S NUTRITION GOAL　　　　　DATE

_____ ☐

WATER DRINKING GOAL　　　　　**EXERCISE GOAL**

_____ ☐　　_____ ☐

TODAY'S MEALS

Planned　　　　　Actual　　　　Calories　　Protein / Carbs / Fat

_____|_____　_____　_____ _____ _____
_____|_____　_____　_____ _____ _____
_____|_____　_____　_____ _____ _____
......................|......................　.......　....... ....
......................|......................　.......　....... ....

SNACKS, DRINKS, & OTHER

_____　_____ _____ _____ _____
_____　_____ _____ _____ _____

TODAY'S TOTALS: _____ _____ _____ _____

BENEFITS I FELT TODAY (CIRCLE):

Feel　　　More　　　Increased　　Improved　　More　　　Reduced
Happier　　Creative　　Willpower　　Focus　　　Energized　　Stress

Day 17: **Pro-Tip**

Make use of vitamins & supplements.

Vitamins are micronutrients that we need for daily functioning. The true end goal of healthy eating is giving your body everything it needs for a long, energy-filled life. Making sure you eat the right amount of vegetables and fruits plays a huge role, but don't be afraid to let vitamins and other natural supplements fill any gaps.

Ask your doctor for recommendations for multi-vitamins and other natural supplements to help ensure your body is getting everything it needs.

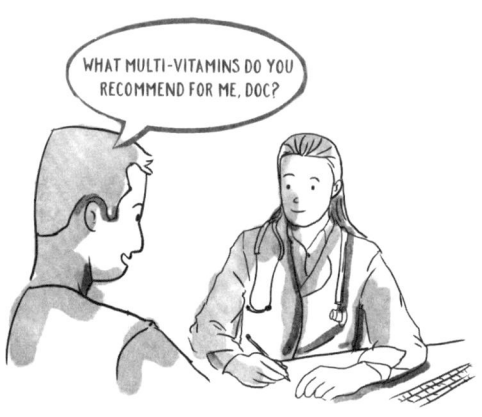

"Don't wait until everything is just right. It will never be perfect. There will always be challenges, obstacles and less than perfect conditions. So what. Get started now. With each step you take, you will grow stronger and stronger, more and more skilled, more and more self-confident and more and more successful."
- Mark Victor Hansen

⊕ **TODAY'S NUTRITION GOAL**   DATE

_____ ☐

◊ **WATER DRINKING GOAL**   🚶 **EXERCISE GOAL**

_____ ☐   _____ ☐

🍴 **TODAY'S MEALS**

Planned	Actual	Calories	Protein / Carbs / Fat

🍎 SNACKS, DRINKS, & OTHER

TODAY'S TOTALS: _____

✓ **BENEFITS I FELT TODAY (CIRCLE):**

Feel Happier | More Creative | Increased Willpower | Improved Focus | More Energized | Reduced Stress

Day 18: **Daily Challenge**

Try meal prepping for a night.

There are lots of advantages to cooking all the meals you plan to eat in the next few days. The main upsides are:

- You save money by cooking in bulk
- You can perfectly track the calories + macronutrients of your food
- It becomes harder to eat foods not part of your eating goals as they are not as readily available
- You save calories as most outside food is cooked with lots of unhealthy oils and butter

For people who have never cooked before, an easy starting point would be to buy pre-cooked foods from a local grocery store that are frozen and simply need to be heated up.

After preparing your food, you can store it in Tupperware then heat it using a microwave when it's time to eat.

There are lots of great resources on YouTube and a whole community dedicated to meal prepping on Instagram (one of our favorites being @meowmeix) you can use for guidance and inspiration as well.

☐ I completed this daily challenge.

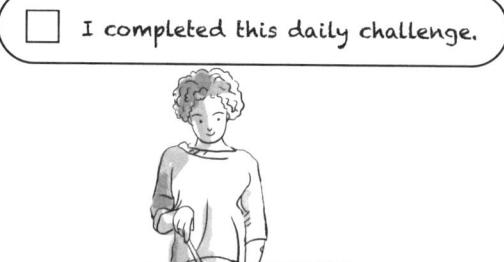

"First we form habits; then they form us. Conquer your bad habits or they will conquer you." - Robert Gilbert

⊕ **TODAY'S NUTRITION GOAL**   DATE

_____ ☐

◊ **WATER DRINKING GOAL**   ⚲ **EXERCISE GOAL**

_____ ☐   _____ ☐

🍽 **TODAY'S MEALS**

| 📅 Planned | ✓ Actual | Calories | Protein / Carbs / Fat |

🍎 SNACKS, DRINKS, & OTHER

TODAY'S TOTALS: _____

✓ **BENEFITS I FELT TODAY (CIRCLE):**

Feel Happier   More Creative   Increased Willpower   Improved Focus   More Energized   Reduced Stress

Day 19: YouTube Alert!

674,000+ SUBSCRIBERS

Clean & delicious.

One of the hardest things about sticking to a healthy eating regimen is making your own food that is both healthy AND tastes good. Dani Spies is a health, wellness and weight loss coach whose mission is to help us all eat better, cook more, and feel great while doing so. She's dedicated to helping people get off the traditional 'diet' and "put you back in the driver seat of your health and body."

Definitely check out her channel for unlimited recipes and healthy food options you can make along with her in the comfort of your own home.

Recommended YouTube Video (search this in YouTube):
Clean & Delicious - Baked Buffalo Cauliflower Bites Recipe

Subscribe here: https://www.youtube.com/user/danispies

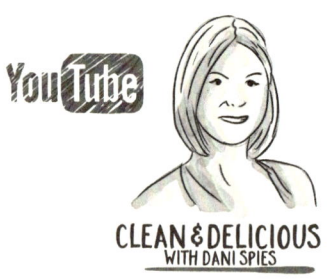

"The road to success is dotted with many tempting parking places."
-Unknown

TODAY'S NUTRITION GOAL

DATE

_____ ☐

WATER DRINKING GOAL **EXERCISE GOAL**

_____ ☐ _____ ☐

TODAY'S MEALS

Planned   Actual   Calories   Protein / Carbs / Fat

_____|_____   _____   _____ _____ _____

_____|_____   _____   _____ _____ _____

_____|_____   _____   _____ _____ _____

...............|...............   ....

...............|...............   ....

SNACKS, DRINKS, & OTHER

_____   _____ _____ _____

_____   _____ _____ _____

TODAY'S TOTALS: _____   _____ _____ _____

BENEFITS I FELT TODAY (CIRCLE):

Feel Happier   More Creative   Increased Willpower   Improved Focus   More Energized   Reduced Stress

Day 20: **Affirmations**

1. Find a quiet area you can do this in private so you can do this at ease. If you can't find a private space, say these in your head while pretending you're screaming it from a mountaintop.

2. Think of a time where you felt absolutely powerful - **where you felt on top of the world.** Tap into every emotion you had at that moment and get yourself into that state right now. How were you feeling then - Powerful? Unstoppable? Strong? Incredible!? Get into it now!!!!

3. Now feel your intensity grow tenfold! Say this with deep passion:

I choose to eat well so that I will feel well. I live healthfully, not only for myself, but also for the people I love, so that they may be empowered to improve their health. Clean, natural foods are a precious gift from the earth, and I thank the earth by eating them abundantly and gratefully. I expect a lot from my body, so I affirm my body's right to expect healthy fuel from me.

Repeat this **one more time.**

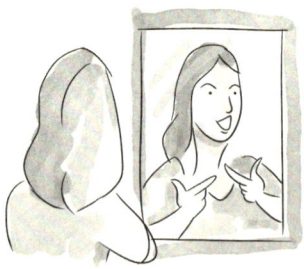

"Whatever course you decide upon, there is always someone to tell you that you are wrong. There are always difficulties arising which tempt you to believe that your critics are right. To map out a course of action and follow it to an end requires courage." - Ralph Waldo Emerson

DATE _____

⊕ **TODAY'S NUTRITION GOAL**

_____ ☐

💧 **WATER DRINKING GOAL**   🚶 **EXERCISE GOAL**

_____ ☐   _____ ☐

🍽 **TODAY'S MEALS**

📅 Planned	✓ Actual	Calories	Protein / Carbs / Fat

🍎 SNACKS, DRINKS, & OTHER

_____   _____

_____   _____

TODAY'S TOTALS: _____ ____ ____

✓ **BENEFITS I FELT TODAY (CIRCLE):**

 Feel Happier   More Creative   Increased Willpower   Improved Focus   More Energized   Reduced Stress

Day 21: **Daily Challenge**

Incorporate more weight & resistance training into your workouts.

It is common to get hooked into how many calories are burned from doing cardio machines like the elliptical or treadmill, especially as they show their estimated calories burned on screen.

Doing cardio is great, but when done in excess it has its downsides as well. Mainly, it can lead an a large slow down of your metabolism, especially when paired with a large caloric deficit - oftentimes doing the opposite of what you wanted initially.

Another big downside is the fact that doing too much cardio with a caloric deficit can lead to losing muscle, which is so important to long-term health.

A Harvard study has shown that **we lose 0.3% to 0.5% of our muscle mass every year, but only if we are not doing progressive weight or resistance training.** This is why you may see older people looking weaker and frail. (https://www.health.harvard.edu/staying-healthy/preserve-your-muscle-mass)

Incorporating muscle/weight training into a weekly workout regimen can help keep you healthy for years to come. Not to mention, the added muscle helps speed up your metabolism, burning more calories throughout each day without extra work.

☐ I completed this daily challenge.

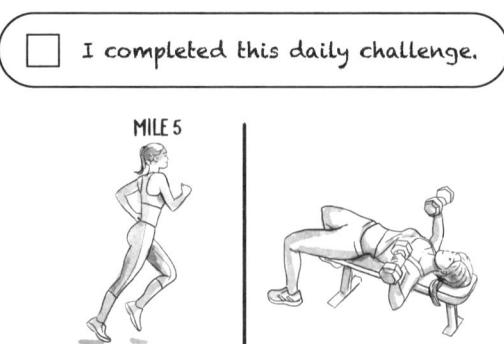

⊕ **TODAY'S NUTRITION GOAL**　　　　　　　DATE

_____ ☐

💧 **WATER DRINKING GOAL**　　　🚶 **EXERCISE GOAL**

_____ ☐　　　_____ ☐

🍴 **TODAY'S MEALS**

📅 Planned　　　　✓ Actual　　　　Calories　　Protein / Carbs / Fat

_____

_____

_____

....

....

🍎 SNACKS, DRINKS, & OTHER

_____

_____

TODAY'S TOTALS: _____

✓ **BENEFITS I FELT TODAY (CIRCLE):**

Feel Happier　More Creative　Increased Willpower　Improved Focus　More Energized　Reduced Stress

~~PHASE 2:~~
DESTROYED.

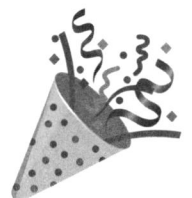 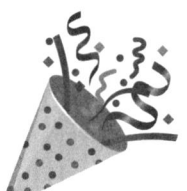 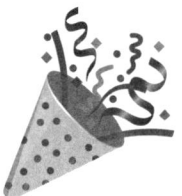

Note: We LOVE sharing stories of our users and what their lives looked like BEFORE using the journal compared to where they are NOW!

If you want to share your story with us, you can do so here:
habitnest.com/nutritiontestimonial

Phase 2 Recap: Days 8-21

1. What have you realized to be the most important elements for you to stick to a healthy eating regimen that will lead to your goal body?

_____

_____

2. What eating habits should you be doing consistently?

_____

_____

3. What are some new strategies you want to experiment with?

_____

_____

4. How has your new healthy eating habit impacted your life?

_____

_____

_____

5. How would you feel if you stopped doing this?

_____

_____

_____

PHASE 3:
DAYS 22-66+

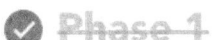 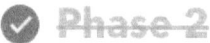 **Phase 3**

~~Days 01-07~~ ~~Days 08-21~~ **Days 22-66+**
~~Hell Week~~ ~~Staying Consistent~~ **Rewiring Your Brain.**

Phase 3: Hardwiring - Retaining Interest in Your Personal Improvement

Congratulations, you've made it to Phase 3. You've shown serious commitment to the incredible future you envision for yourself.

Now, it's about making sure you continue to love the benefits you've been seeing, remain consistent, and maintain the interest you began this whole journey with.

It's easy to take the benefits you're feeling for granted -it's extremely easy to fall off the wagon, especially in this phase.

Keep going strong until healthy eating is engrained in your DNA.

This means pushing through to stick with your commitments on your best days, your worst days, and especially the days you just don't feel like it (those are the *most important*).

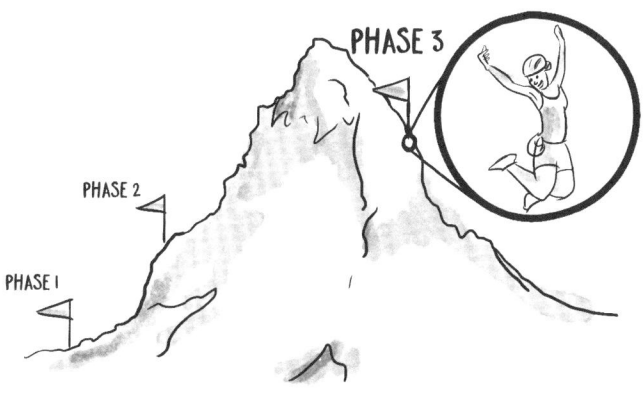

Commit.

I am INCREDIBLE.

*I've come a long way,
but the road doesn't end here.*

It's time to ingrain this habit in me forever.

*I will see this
huge challenge all the way through.*

*Mastering this habit is only the
beginning of my perpetual growth.*

_____

Nothing will stop me now.

_____   _____
Signature   Date

Day 22: **Pro-Tip**

Keep it simple.

The more simple your food is (i.e. the less ingredients in your food), the more you know about it. The more you know about what your food consists of, the easier it is to gain knowledge about how different types of food affect your body.

Start thinking of yourself as a scientist and do your best to see how different foods affect your energy levels, which foods make you feel more or less satiated, and even whether they affect your mood.

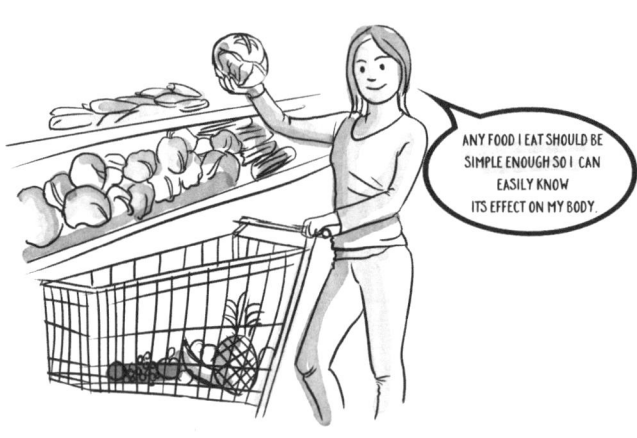

"The easier it is to do, the harder it is to change."
- Eng's Principle

TODAY'S NUTRITION GOAL

DATE _____

_____ ☐

💧 WATER DRINKING GOAL 🚶 EXERCISE GOAL

_____ ☐   _____ ☐

🍽 TODAY'S MEALS

| 📋 Planned | ✓ Actual | Calories | Protein / Carbs / Fat |

🍎 SNACKS, DRINKS, & OTHER

TODAY'S TOTALS: _____

HOW DID MY EATING CHOICES IMPACT MY DAY?

_____
_____
_____
_____

Day 23: **Daily Challenge**

Challenge: Party smart.

Special events should be a very important thing to consider, especially if you consistently attend more than one event per month. The next time you have one, prepare for it as much as possible during the day as it is so easy to overeat.

One approach is to save room during the day with smaller meals to create room for eating more at night without breaking your goals.

Alternatively, if you know you will overeat if you are starving, have a pre-party snack and tons of water. **Dehydration is a big reason that leads to overeating** and can be easily avoided if you come thoroughly prepared.

At the event, avoid the food pile-up at the buffet. Choose the smallest plate, do not stack your food, and make sure there is space between each food item. You must be able to see everything on your plate clearly.

Going to a special event can be like going to war - be as ready as possible.

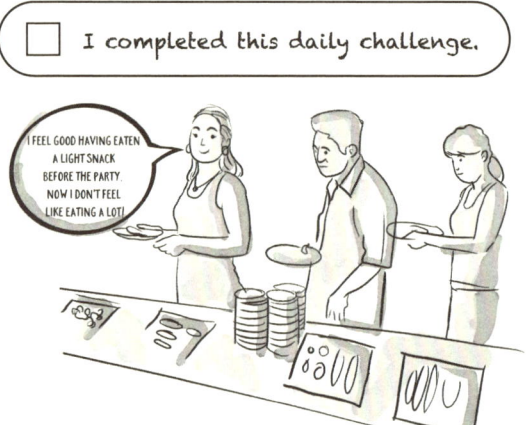

"I tried every diet in the book. I tried some that weren't in the book. I tried eating the book. It tasted better than most of the diets." - Dolly Parton

TODAY'S NUTRITION GOAL

DATE _____

_____ ☐

WATER DRINKING GOAL

EXERCISE GOAL

_____ ☐   _____ ☐

TODAY'S MEALS

Planned	Actual	Calories	Protein / Carbs / Fat

SNACKS, DRINKS, & OTHER

TODAY'S TOTALS: _____

HOW DID MY EATING CHOICES IMPACT MY DAY?

_____

_____

_____

_____

Day 24: **Affirmations**

1. Find a quiet area where you can do this in private so you can do this at ease. If you can't find a private space, say these in your head while pretending you're screaming them from a mountaintop.

2. Think of a time where you felt absolutely powerful - **where you felt on top of the world**. Tap into every emotion you had at that moment and get yourself into that state right now. How were you feeling then - Powerful? Unstoppable? Strong? Incredible!? Get into it now!!!!

3. Now feel your intensity grow tenfold! Say this with deep passion:

I do not overeat because I know my body doesn't want to have to signal to me that it is overfull. Eating healthfully is empowering and gives me full control of my wellness. I am the only person who has control over my eating habits, and I can always resist unhealthy foods if I choose to.

Repeat this **one more time**.

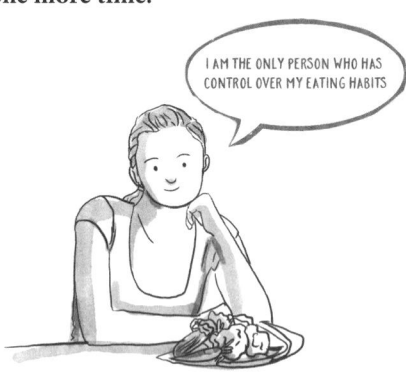

"Affirmations are like seed planted in soil. Poor soil, poor growth. Rich soil, abundant growth. The more you choose to think thoughts that make you feel good, the quicker the affirmations work."
- Louise L. Hay

TODAY'S NUTRITION GOAL

DATE _____

_____ ☐

WATER DRINKING GOAL

EXERCISE GOAL

_____ ☐   _____ ☐

TODAY'S MEALS

Planned	Actual	Calories	Protein / Carbs / Fat
....	....		
....	....		

SNACKS, DRINKS, & OTHER

_____

_____

TODAY'S TOTALS: _____

HOW DID MY EATING CHOICES IMPACT MY DAY?

_____

_____

_____

_____

Day 25: **Super Read**

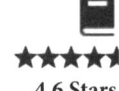

Title: *In Defense of Food: An Eater's Manifesto*   4.6 Stars

Author: Michael Pollan
Note: We have no affiliation with Pollan or his works, we simply think his book is a great resource.

Michael Pollan is THE expert on food. If you want to understand exactly how to be healthy, this book is an absolute must read. To sum up his thoughts in a few words, "Eat food. Not too much. Mostly plants."

He also has an amazing documentary on Netflix titled *In Defense of Food* which outlines his philosophy and literally goes through the history of how our ideas about macronutrients is in a constant state of change. He might in fact be the most well-versed healthy eating expert on the planet.

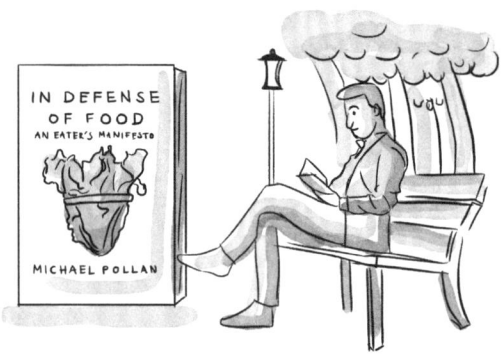

"The cardiologist's diet: If it tastes good, spit it out."
- Unknown

TODAY'S NUTRITION GOAL

DATE

_____ ☐

WATER DRINKING GOAL   EXERCISE GOAL

_____ ☐   _____ ☐

TODAY'S MEALS

Planned   Actual   Calories   Protein / Carbs / Fat

SNACKS, DRINKS, & OTHER

TODAY'S TOTALS: _____

HOW DID MY EATING CHOICES IMPACT MY DAY?

_____

_____

_____

_____

Day 26: **Daily Challenge**

Challenge: Drink one gallon of water!

Yes, one entire gallon. We underestimate the value and potential benefits drinking a lot of water can have on our bodies because we don't do it consistently enough to see how big of a difference it'll make.

A gallon of water can help us lose weight by reducing hunger, increasing our metabolism, aiding in digestion and preventing constipation. On top of all that, it's the best remedy for headaches, makes us feel fresh throughout the day, boosts our immune systems, improves skin health and increases our energy levels.

Superhero option: For one week, commit to drinking one gallon of water a day no matter how hard the first few days are. Carry a bottle with you. Make rules for when you'll drink, like every time you get up from your seat, every time you sit back down, as soon as you wake up, every time you go to the restroom, etc. If you complete this challenge you'll forget what life was like before consistently drinking water!

☐ I completed this daily challenge.

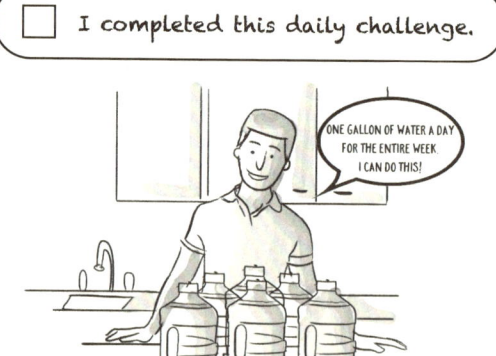

"My advice if you insist on slimming: Eat as much as you like – just don't swallow it." - Harry Secombe

TODAY'S NUTRITION GOAL　　　　　　　　DATE

_____ ☐

WATER DRINKING GOAL　　　　**EXERCISE GOAL**

_____ ☐　　_____ ☐

TODAY'S MEALS

Planned	Actual	Calories	Protein / Carbs / Fat

SNACKS, DRINKS, & OTHER

_____

_____

TODAY'S TOTALS: _____ _____

HOW DID MY EATING CHOICES IMPACT MY DAY?

_____

_____

_____

Day 27: **Pro-Tip**

Do NOT do diet soda.

Studies conducted at the University of Texas Health Science Center and Purdue University have shed light on whether diet soda actually helps us lose weight. They found that one to two cans of diet soda daily can actually increase our waistlines by up to 500% because artificial sweeteners actually interrupt the body's ability to regulate our calorie intake. Also, sugar makes us crave sugar. When we're drinking diet sodas, our body thinks it's getting sugar, which causes it to crave more, which naturally leads to over-eating of the wrong types of foods.

Diet soda is also linked to increased risk of metabolic syndrome - a group of adverse medical conditions that increase one's risk of heart disease.

So don't make the mistake of thinking that zero-calorie drinks are helping you lose weight. Do your best to avoid drinks with sugar, and drinks with fake sugar.

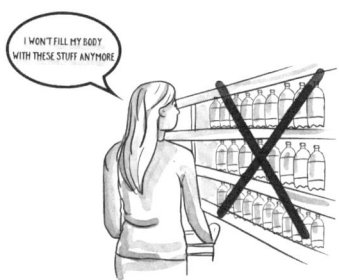

"A diet is a plan, generally hopeless, for reducing your weight, which tests your will power but does little for your waistline."
- Herbert B. Prochnow

TODAY'S NUTRITION GOAL DATE

_____ ☐

WATER DRINKING GOAL   **EXERCISE GOAL**

_____ ☐   _____ ☐

TODAY'S MEALS

Planned   Actual   Calories   Protein / Carbs / Fat

SNACKS, DRINKS, & OTHER

TODAY'S TOTALS: _____

HOW DID MY EATING CHOICES IMPACT MY DAY?

Day 28: **Affirmations**

1. Find a quiet area where you can do this in private so you can do this at ease. If you can't find a private space, say these in your head while pretending you're screaming them from a mountaintop.

2. Think of a time where you felt absolutely powerful - **where you felt on top of the world**. Tap into every emotion you had at that moment and get yourself into that state right now. How were you feeling then - Powerful? Unstoppable? Strong? Incredible!? Get into it now!!!!

3. Now feel your intensity grow tenfold! Say this with deep passion:

I pay close attention to where my food comes from and I think deeply about the resources that go into each meal. I am mindful to eat as much as I can from what the earth naturally gives me. My body has the right to receive what will make it feel good, and when I feed it healthy foods, I am amazed at how well my body works.

Repeat this **one more time.**

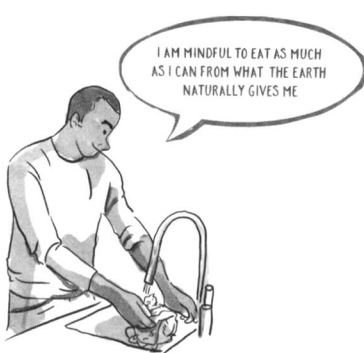

"Don't let the fear of the time it will take to accomplish something stand in the way of your doing it. The time will pass anyway; we might as well put that passing time to the best possible use." - Earl Nightingale

TODAY'S NUTRITION GOAL　　　　　　　　　　　DATE

_____　☐

WATER DRINKING GOAL　　　　**EXERCISE GOAL**

_____　☐　_____　☐

TODAY'S MEALS

Planned	Actual	Calories	Protein / Carbs / Fat

SNACKS, DRINKS, & OTHER

TODAY'S TOTALS: _____

HOW DID MY EATING CHOICES IMPACT MY DAY?

_____
_____
_____
_____

Progress Tracker (Optional)

Progress Picture (Front)

Progress Picture (Side)

How happy am I with myself (circle one)?

1   2   3   4   5

Previous Weight	Previous Body Fat %
Weight	Body Fat %

Day 29: Favorite Podcasts

No Meat Athlete Radio.

iTunes Reviews: 720
★★★★★ 4.5

It's no secret that a largely plant-based diet will generally lead to weight loss, but what other benefits does it provide? Can we really get all the energy and protein we need without chicken or other meat? Host Matt Frazier gives a voice to plant-powered jocks. He's not about getting you to change who you are. He just wants to provide anyone with training tips, recipes, a discussion of the benefits, and inspiration to anyone who wants to lose weight and is considering a more plant-based approach to their diet.

How to get started:

1. Find the podcast "No Meat Athlete Radio" and choose an episode to listen to.
2. Download the episode to your phone.
3. Go in airplane mode and play the episode.
4. Set your podcast player to automatically stop after the current episode finishes. You can do this on iOS by hitting the moon icon on the bottom of the podcast page (while an episode is playing) and selecting the time you want it to stop playing.

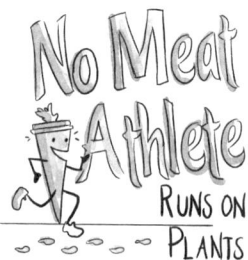

"Sugar is A problem in the average diet. But it's not THE problem."
-Catherine Saxelby

⊕ **TODAY'S NUTRITION GOAL** DATE

◊ **WATER DRINKING GOAL** 　　🚶 **EXERCISE GOAL**

🍴 **TODAY'S MEALS**

📅 Planned	✓ Actual	Calories	Protein / Carbs / Fat

🍎 SNACKS, DRINKS, & OTHER

TODAY'S TOTALS: _____

HOW DID MY EATING CHOICES IMPACT MY DAY?

Day 30: **Pro-Tip**

Audit your calorie counting to find potential mistakes.

If you are counting calories, there will **always** be a layer of inaccuracy. This is okay - though our goal is to lower that inaccuracy as much as possible and to stay consistent with counting over time.

Check to see which of these you may occasionally be missing:

- **Not counting low calorie foods** like veggies.

- **Not counting oils/butter** that are used in the cooking process.

- **Underestimating the calories in an outside meal**. On average they have more calories because of oils used, so be extra careful!

- **Not counting little bites of things** you have throughout the day. Count them, even if they're small like 10-25 calories for each. You can add them to your snacks section in the journal.

- **Not trusting the science of the counting process.** It's common to think our bodies are naturally "different" when we don't see the results we want, when really we are making a mistake somewhere in our tracking. This process only works if you respect and play by its rules, accepting any times you veer off course open-heartedly.

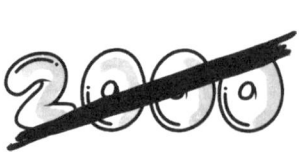 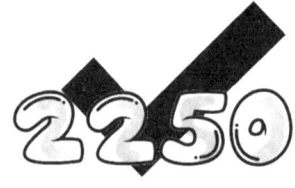

"It's not who you think you are that holds you back; it's who you think you're not." - Unknown

TODAY'S NUTRITION GOAL

DATE

_____ ☐

WATER DRINKING GOAL **EXERCISE GOAL**

_____ ☐ _____ ☐

TODAY'S MEALS

Planned | Actual | Calories | Protein / Carbs / Fat

SNACKS, DRINKS, & OTHER

TODAY'S TOTALS: _____

HOW DID MY EATING CHOICES IMPACT MY DAY?

_____
_____
_____
_____

Day 31: **Affirmations**

1. Find a quiet area where you can do this in private so you can do this at ease. If you can't find a private space, say these in your head while pretending you're screaming them from a mountaintop.

2. Think of a time where you felt absolutely powerful - **where you felt on top of the world**. Tap into every emotion you had at that moment and get yourself into that state right now. How were you feeling then - Powerful? Unstoppable? Strong? Incredible!? Get into it now!!!!

3. Now feel your intensity grow tenfold! Say this with deep passion:

I no longer eat when I am not hungry and I can easily deny foods that I know will cause my body to feel indigestion and discomfort.

I refuse to eat with my eyes; rather, I eat what my body communicates to me that it needs.

Repeat this **one more time**.

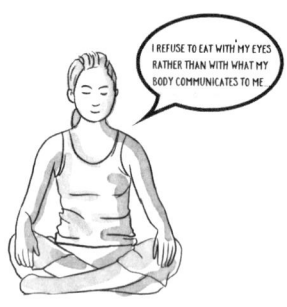

"Negative results are just what I want. They're just as valuable to me as positive results. I can never find the thing that does the job best until I find the ones that don't."
- Thomas Edison

TODAY'S NUTRITION GOAL DATE

☐

WATER DRINKING GOAL   **EXERCISE GOAL**

☐   ☐

TODAY'S MEALS

Planned   Actual   Calories   Protein / Carbs / Fat

SNACKS, DRINKS, & OTHER

TODAY'S TOTALS: _____

HOW DID MY EATING CHOICES IMPACT MY DAY?

Day 32: **Pro-Tip**

Creative ways to satisfy your sweet tooth cravings.

Sweet food is DELICIOUS, and hunger cravings for them can sometimes feel so great to give in to, though they set us back very far on our goals. Here are some alternatives you can use to get over your sweet tooth cravings:

1. **Eat your berries!** Strawberries, blueberries, raspberries, blackberries, boysenberries, among others, are some of the best snacks to eat regularly and can help satisfy your sweet tooth. You can also try freezing your berries (or grapes!)

2. If you have an undying need to eat chocolate, **break a piece of dark chocolate off**, take it to another room, and let small pieces melt in your mouth (no chewing!) This can give you a few minutes of sweetness in your mouth for a lot less calories.

3. **Use See's Candies™ Lollypops** (no affiliation). These are available online at most retail outlets, have roughly ~90 calories, and can take 10-30 minutes to finish, satisfying your taste for having something sweet in your mouth for a very long time.

4. **Eat some coconut oil!** Although very high in calories (~100 per tbsp), it is incredibly effective at removing sweet tooth cravings.

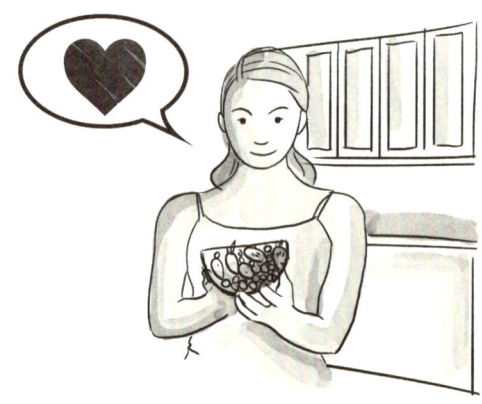

TODAY'S NUTRITION GOAL

DATE

_____ ☐

WATER DRINKING GOAL   **EXERCISE GOAL**

_____ ☐   _____ ☐

TODAY'S MEALS

Planned	Actual	Calories	Protein / Carbs / Fat

SNACKS, DRINKS, & OTHER

TODAY'S TOTALS: _____

HOW DID MY EATING CHOICES IMPACT MY DAY?

_____
_____
_____
_____

Day 33: **Pro-Tip**

Maintaining can be more difficult than losing.

As you progress on this journey of health and fat loss, there is one critically important thing to keep in mind. Losing weight can be really difficult, but maintaining your results is arguably more difficult.

Our hope for you isn't to help you lose weight, feel really good for a few months, and then fall right back into old habits.

Our wish is that you take this learning process really seriously, make one small change at a time, see consistent results, and ultimately incorporate a healthier diet as part of your overall lifestyle because you love the way it makes you feel about yourself.

You need just as much discipline to maintain your progress as you do to get to your goal.

One helpful way to incorporate this knowledge into your mindset is to think of your goal not as simply achieving a certain weight or percentage of fat loss, but rather making your goal achieving a certain weight AND maintaining that weight for the next 6 months.

Because in reality, your goal is to have these results forever!

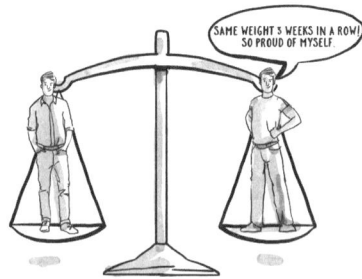

"Nothing will work unless you do." - Maya Angelou

TODAY'S NUTRITION GOAL

_____ ☐

DATE _____

WATER DRINKING GOAL

_____ ☐

EXERCISE GOAL

_____ ☐

TODAY'S MEALS

Planned	Actual	Calories	Protein / Carbs / Fat

SNACKS, DRINKS, & OTHER

_____

_____

TODAY'S TOTALS: _____ _____ _____ _____

HOW DID MY EATING CHOICES IMPACT MY DAY?

_____

_____

_____

_____

Day 34: **Success Story**

Zach Galifinakis.
Actor, writer & comedian; Lost 50 lbs

Many know Zach Galifinakis as the hilariously chubby 'Allen' from the hangover. What most people don't know is that in 2012 he lost about 50 pounds by simply cutting alcohol from his diet and walking more often. When asked about the transformation he's said, "I stopped drinking and I just kind of put the weight off, I was having a lot of vodka with sausage. Delicious but bad for you."

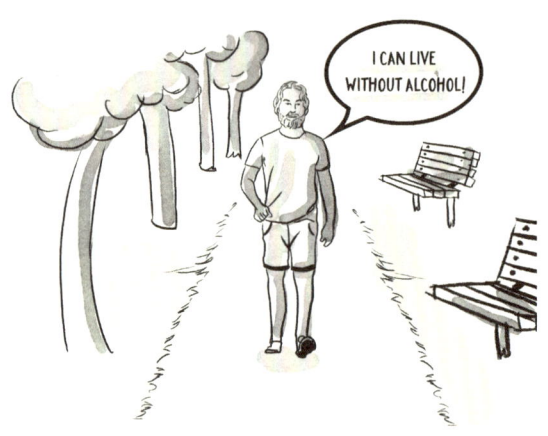

"The starting point of all achievement is desire. Keep this constantly in mind. Weak desires bring weak results, just as a small amount of fire makes a small amount of heat."
- Napoleon Hill

TODAY'S NUTRITION GOAL   DATE
_____ ☐

WATER DRINKING GOAL   **EXERCISE GOAL**
_____ ☐   _____ ☐

TODAY'S MEALS

Planned	Actual	Calories	Protein / Carbs / Fat

SNACKS, DRINKS, & OTHER
_____
_____

TODAY'S TOTALS: _____ ____ ____ ____

HOW DID MY EATING CHOICES IMPACT MY DAY?
_____
_____
_____
_____

Day 35: **Affirmations**

1. Find a quiet area where you can do this in private so you can do this at ease. If you can't find a private space, say these in your head while pretending you're screaming them from a mountaintop.

2. Think of a time where you felt absolutely powerful - **where you felt on top of the world**. Tap into every emotion you had at that moment and get yourself into that state right now. How were you feeling then - Powerful? Unstoppable? Strong? Incredible!? Get into it now!!!!

3. Now feel your intensity grow tenfold! Say this with deep passion:

When I eat, I enjoy every single bite. I realize that being able to choose what I eat is a luxury not everyone can afford. I not only enjoy my food, but I willingly choose to eat what I know will make me feel good, inside and out.

Repeat this **one more time.**

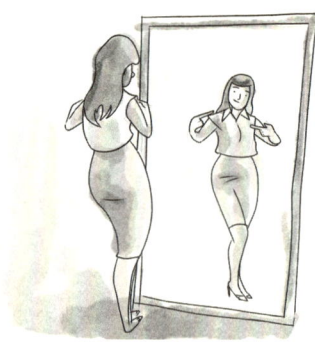

"You have to put in many, many, many tiny efforts that nobody sees or appreciates before you achieve anything worthwhile."
- Brian Tracy

TODAY'S NUTRITION GOAL　　　　　　　DATE

_____　☐

WATER DRINKING GOAL　　　　**EXERCISE GOAL**

_____ ☐　　_____ ☐

TODAY'S MEALS

Planned	Actual	Calories	Protein / Carbs / Fat

SNACKS, DRINKS, & OTHER

TODAY'S TOTALS: _____

HOW DID MY EATING CHOICES IMPACT MY DAY?

_____
_____
_____
_____

Day 36: **Success Story**

Melissa McCarthy.
Actress, comedian, fashion designer, producer; Lost 75 lbs

Melissa McCarthy is kind of like the female version of Zach Galifinakis from The Hangover - absolutely hilarious and overweight. Not anymore! At 46 she's lost over 75 pounds. When asked about the transformation, she's jokingly said, "I cried off the pounds." Ha. She actually attributes her success to not stressing and worrying so much about her diet. "I truly stopped worrying about it. I think there's something to kinda loosening up and not being so nervous and rigid about it that, bizarrely, has worked."

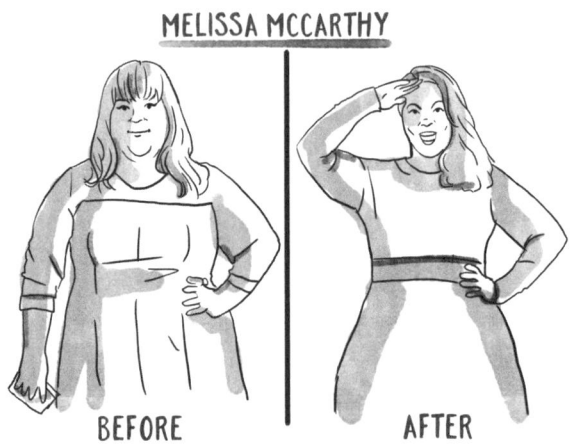

"Do what you have to do until you can do what you want to do."
—Oprah Winfrey

TODAY'S NUTRITION GOAL

DATE

WATER DRINKING GOAL

EXERCISE GOAL

TODAY'S MEALS

Planned | Actual | Calories | Protein / Carbs / Fat

SNACKS, DRINKS, & OTHER

TODAY'S TOTALS: _____

HOW DID MY EATING CHOICES IMPACT MY DAY?

Day 37: **Daily Challenge**

Challenge: Think about what the image of perfection you've created for yourself is... Now realize that you may NEVER fit that image! Instead, be yourself and love yourself for all that you are.

Most of us subconsciously judge ourselves for not fitting this image of perfection whenever we slip up or struggle, even the slightest bit. This is a horrendous activity that will lead you to unhappiness, a spiral of guilt, a feeling of unworthiness, and freeze you in inactivity.

What does this cycle do to help you succeed and live a happy life? **NOTHING**. The truth is, the quicker you can do the following, the happier your life will be day after day.

Whenever you feel you're not in a state of pure happiness:

1. Determine what mistakes you made and what went wrong.
2. Identify what you can learn from these mistakes and apply it to your future.
3. **Forgive yourself.** Now forgive yourself again.
4. Love yourself for exactly who you are right now.
5. Now **move forward full speed ahead** with what you've learned.

It doesn't matter if it takes you 50 learning cycles or 5 years of mistakes - the second you lose is when you throw on that useless guilt and those unnecessary negative emotions because you're trashing your quality of life... and increasing your quality of life is the whole point you're doing this in the first place!

☐ I completed this daily challenge.

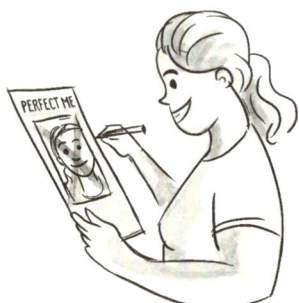

TODAY'S NUTRITION GOAL

DATE

WATER DRINKING GOAL

EXERCISE GOAL

TODAY'S MEALS

Planned	Actual	Calories	Protein / Carbs / Fat

SNACKS, DRINKS, & OTHER

TODAY'S TOTALS: _____

HOW DID MY EATING CHOICES IMPACT MY DAY?

Day 38: **Favorite Resources** 🔧

Product: Accu-Measure body fat caliper.
Cost: $10
Note: We have no affiliation with Accu-Measure. We just love the tool.

If one of your core nutrition goals is to improve your body composition, just using a scale and/or the mirror is an ineffective way to track your progress.

This is especially useful if you also want to build more muscle, as you'll be able to get a much better idea if you are gaining muscle and/or losing fat instead of just seeing weight fluctuations on a scale.

The Accu-Measure can be very accurate (they ran a study that showed 98% accuracy compared to water displacement tests). However, one downside to be weary of is it is only accurate if you are using it both consistently and accurately - which is not the most straightforward thing to do. We give some tips on how to bypass this in the intro section of this book if it interests you.

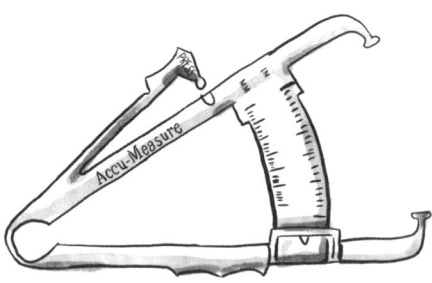

"A dream doesn't become reality through magic; it takes sweat, determination and hard work. The price of success is hard work, dedication to the job at hand, and the determination that whether we win or lose, we have applied the best of ourselves to the task at hand."
- Vince Lombardi

TODAY'S NUTRITION GOAL   DATE

_____ ☐

WATER DRINKING GOAL   **EXERCISE GOAL**

_____ ☐   _____ ☐

TODAY'S MEALS

Planned   Actual   Calories   Protein / Carbs / Fat

SNACKS, DRINKS, & OTHER

TODAY'S TOTALS: _____

HOW DID MY EATING CHOICES IMPACT MY DAY?

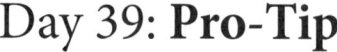

Day 39: **Pro-Tip**

Your kitchen tells the future.

You can't expect to eat healthy at home if your kitchen isn't filled with what you need. If the fridge and pantry are packed with ice cream, cookies, beer and bacon… it's just not going to work.

If you do the shopping in your home, stay conscious of how your shopping will affect your diet. Let your goals guide you, even if you shop for more than just yourself. If you're not the home shopper, at the very least, request healthy foods from whomever shops for the home and ask that they support you in your healthy eating goals.

No matter what you buy, always ALSO get veggies, fruits, lean meats, whole grains, nuts and berries.

Life Hack: Sticking to the outer edges of the grocery store helps you see all the healthy food options available.

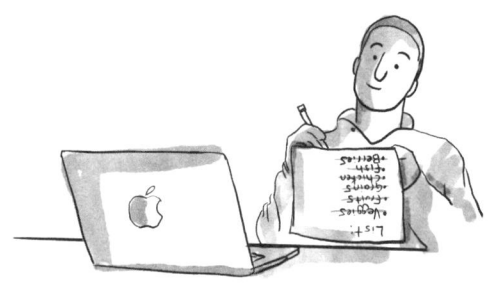

"Weight loss can change your whole character. That always amazed me: Shedding pounds does change your personality. It changes your philosophy of life because you recognize that you are capable of using your mind to change your body." - Jean Nidetch

TODAY'S NUTRITION GOAL

DATE

_____

WATER DRINKING GOAL   EXERCISE GOAL

_____   _____

TODAY'S MEALS

Planned	Actual	Calories	Protein / Carbs / Fat

SNACKS, DRINKS, & OTHER

_____

_____

TODAY'S TOTALS: _____

HOW DID MY EATING CHOICES IMPACT MY DAY?

_____

_____

_____

_____

Day 40: **Daily Challenge**

Challenge: Think deeply about the direct relationship between the actions you take today and your future.

Newsflash: You are exactly a compilation of your past actions. The future version of you is exactly a compilation of the actions you take starting today.

How do you envision yourself in the future? Thin? Confident? Happy with your body? What actions have you taken in the last month that are in direct relation to the future version of yourself you are envisioning?

One of the problems is that we believe in the possibility of a future version of ourselves that's different from who we are in this moment. We imagine that the future version of us will magically begin to take the actions towards the goals we have today, without us altering our actions today.

Our brains function off our habits. Our habits function off our actions. Our actions can only come from from the present moment.

Understand that our dream lives only exist if we change our behaviors TODAY.

☐ I completed this daily challenge.

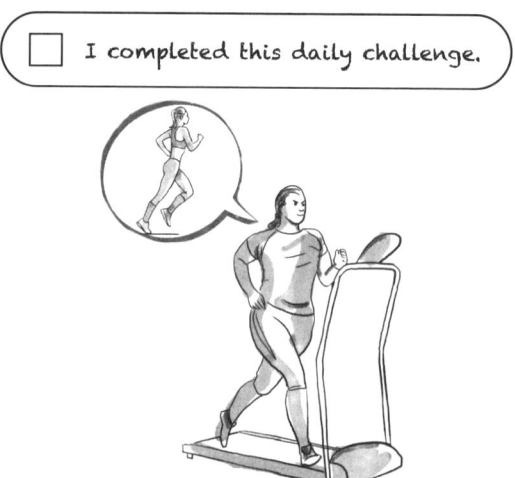

TODAY'S NUTRITION GOAL

DATE: _____

_____ ☐

WATER DRINKING GOAL

_____ ☐

EXERCISE GOAL

_____ ☐

TODAY'S MEALS

Planned	Actual	Calories	Protein / Carbs / Fat

SNACKS, DRINKS, & OTHER

TODAY'S TOTALS: _____

HOW DID MY EATING CHOICES IMPACT MY DAY?

_____
_____
_____
_____

Day 41: Pro-Tip

Chew, a lot.

Proper digestion and nutrient absorption starts with chewing your food an appropriate amount. Properly chewing your food reduces stress on your esophagus and allows. your stomach to easily metabolize your food.

Obviously, different types of food require different amounts of chewing. Research conducted at Ohio State University has found that chewing softer foods 5-10 times before swallowing works well, and 20-30 times for denser foods like meat and vegetables.

This will also help give your body time to communicate to your brain that you're full, so you're at less risk of over-eating, especially when you're really hungry.

WHEN YOU BIT OFF

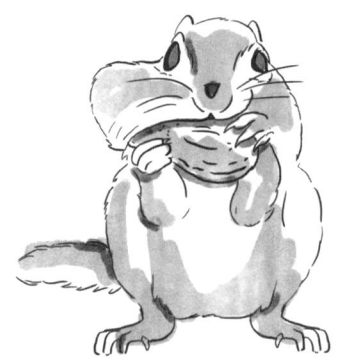

MORE THAN YOU COULD CHEW

"Inside some of us is a thin person struggling to get out, but they can usually be sedated with a few pieces of chocolate cake."
- Unknown

TODAY'S NUTRITION GOAL　　　DATE

_____ ☐

WATER DRINKING GOAL　　　**EXERCISE GOAL**

_____ ☐　_____ ☐

TODAY'S MEALS

Planned	Actual	Calories	Protein / Carbs / Fat

SNACKS, DRINKS, & OTHER

_____

_____

TODAY'S TOTALS: _____ ____ ____ ____

HOW DID MY EATING CHOICES IMPACT MY DAY?

_____
_____
_____
_____

Day 42: **Favorite Podcasts**

Sound Bites.

iTunes Reviews: 85
★★★★★ 5

When you're ready to get beyond the simple tips and tricks to stick to a healthy eating routine, the *Sound Bites* podcast can help you better understand the science behind nutrition and healthy eating. The host is Melissa Joy Dobbins, a registered dietician and best-selling author who interviews experts, researchers and academics in nutrition, agriculture, and health. She really is one of your go-to authorities on health, weight-management and smart nutrition.

Check out her podcast on *iTunes, iHeart Radio, Stitcher*, or *Spreaker*. To find it you can simply search "Sound Bites RD".

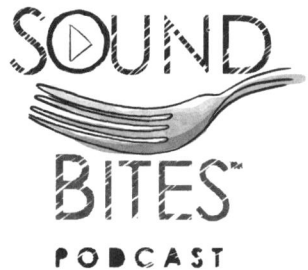

"People are so worried about what they eat between Christmas and the New Year, but they really should be worried about what they eat between the New Year and Christmas."
- Unknown

TODAY'S NUTRITION GOAL DATE

_____ ☐

WATER DRINKING GOAL   **EXERCISE GOAL**

_____ ☐ _____ ☐

TODAY'S MEALS

Planned	Actual	Calories	Protein / Carbs / Fat

SNACKS, DRINKS, & OTHER

TODAY'S TOTALS: _____

HOW DID MY EATING CHOICES IMPACT MY DAY?

_____
_____
_____
_____

Progress Tracker (Optional)

```
┌─────────────────────┐   ┌─────────────────────┐
│                     │   │                     │
│                     │   │                     │
│   Progress Picture  │   │   Progress Picture  │
│       (Front)       │   │       (Side)        │
│                     │   │                     │
│                     │   │                     │
└─────────────────────┘   └─────────────────────┘
```

How happy am I with myself (circle one)?

1   2   3   4   5

_____   _____
Previous Weight   Previous Body Fat %

_____   _____
Weight   Body Fat %

Day 43: **Affirmations**

1. Find a quiet area where you can do this in private so you can do this at ease. If you can't find a private space, say these in your head while pretending you're screaming them from a mountaintop.

2. Think of a time where you felt absolutely powerful - **where you felt on top of the world**. Tap into every emotion you had at that moment and get yourself into that state right now. How were you feeling then - Powerful? Unstoppable? Strong? Incredible!? Get into it now!!!!

3. Now feel your intensity grow tenfold! Say this with deep passion:

When I drink water over less healthy drinks I can feel my body growing hydrated and energetic. When I choose vegetables and fruits over unhealthy snacks, I feel my willpower growing and my body being fueled with what it truly craves. I am the master of my body, and I choose to fill my body with the vitamins and nutrients it deserves.

Repeat this **one more time.**

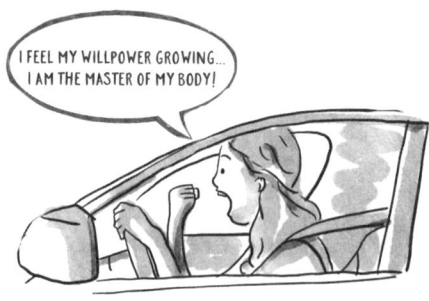

"I keep trying to lose weight... but it keeps finding me."
- Unknown

TODAY'S NUTRITION GOAL

DATE

WATER DRINKING GOAL

EXERCISE GOAL

TODAY'S MEALS

Planned	Actual	Calories	Protein / Carbs / Fat

SNACKS, DRINKS, & OTHER

TODAY'S TOTALS: _____

HOW DID MY EATING CHOICES IMPACT MY DAY?

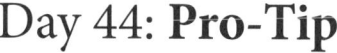

Day 44: **Pro-Tip**

Some amazing food replacement options.

1. Switch out the rice for quinoa
- Quinoa has a ton of protein in it and much more fiber than rice.

2. Switch out the mayo for mustard or hummus
 - Mayo has sugar and saturated fat in it, mustard doesn't.
 - Hummus has a fourth of the calories per tbsp. For a kick, use hummus mixed with Sriracha sauce.

3. Switch out the vegetable oil for coconut or avocado oil
- The fat in coconut oil is much healthier and can support weight loss

4. Use popcorn instead of potato chips
- Popcorn has way less calories and fat, and still feels like junk food

Every small change adds up over time. If you eat a lot of butter, you can lose 10-15 pounds in a year by just cutting butter out of your diet. If you start making these small changes, you WILL see the results add up quickly.

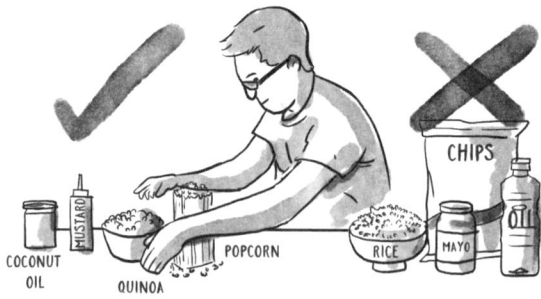

"Keep your dreams alive. Understand to achieve anything requires faith and belief in yourself, vision, hard work, determination, and dedication. Remember all things are possible for those who believe."
- Gail Devers

TODAY'S NUTRITION GOAL　　　　　　　　　DATE

_____ ☐

WATER DRINKING GOAL　　　　**EXERCISE GOAL**

_____ ☐　　_____ ☐

TODAY'S MEALS

Planned　　　　　Actual　　　　Calories　　Protein / Carbs / Fat

SNACKS, DRINKS, & OTHER

TODAY'S TOTALS: _____

HOW DID MY EATING CHOICES IMPACT MY DAY?

_____
_____
_____
_____

Day 45: **Affirmations**

1. Find a quiet area where you can do this in private so you can do this at ease. If you can't find a private space, say these in your head while pretending you're screaming them from a mountaintop.

2. Think of a time where you felt absolutely powerful - **where you felt on top of the world**. Tap into every emotion you had at that moment and get yourself into that state right now. How were you feeling then - Powerful? Unstoppable? Strong? Incredible!? Get into it now!!!!

3. Now feel your intensity grow tenfold! Say this with deep passion:

I choose to change my eating habits, and I successfully do so. I ignore false messages of hunger and eat only when necessary. I love my life and I am immune to the temptation of eating unhealthy foods. I can easily replace the unhealthy foods I eat with natural foods that will nourish my body and provide me with long-lasting energy.

Repeat this **one more time.**

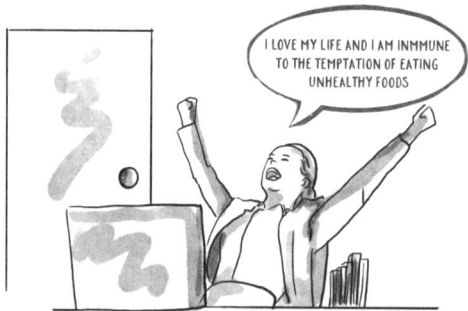

"I've come to believe that all my past failure and frustration were actually laying the foundation for the understandings that have created the new level of living I now enjoy." - Anthony Robbins

TODAY'S NUTRITION GOAL

DATE

☐

WATER DRINKING GOAL   EXERCISE GOAL

☐   ☐

TODAY'S MEALS

Planned	Actual	Calories	Protein / Carbs / Fat

SNACKS, DRINKS, & OTHER

TODAY'S TOTALS: _____

HOW DID MY EATING CHOICES IMPACT MY DAY?

Day 46: **Favorite Resources**
Use a food tracking app alongside your journal.

Although this journal has a built-in calorie/macronutrient counter, one downside is there is no readily available library of foods to use. There are many apps out there with a full database of foods that should cover the majority of what we eat in a day.

Our favorite one is Lifesum (no affiliation) due to the beautiful user interface. You can still use the journal to track your meals and to serve as your guide throughout your healthy eating journey, using it in conjunction with Lifesum (or another app) to help you do the more monotonous parts like calorie/macronutrient tracking. Another commonly used alternative is MyFitnessPal.

This approach can also be useful as you can track foods on the go if you do not have your journal with you, then summarize it at the end of your day in your *Nutrition Sidekick Journal*.

A downside of these apps is they can have inaccuracies for food values (as a lot of the info is user-inputted), so keeping an eye out is important. They can also block some user functionality by forcing you to pay for them or pay for a subscription, so it may end up costing more than expected.

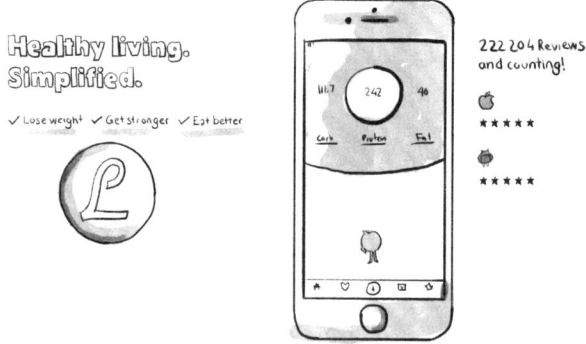

"Man is free at the moment he wishes to be." - Voltaire

TODAY'S NUTRITION GOAL DATE

_____ ☐

WATER DRINKING GOAL   **EXERCISE GOAL**

_____ ☐   _____ ☐

TODAY'S MEALS

Planned   Actual   Calories   Protein / Carbs / Fat

SNACKS, DRINKS, & OTHER

TODAY'S TOTALS: _____

HOW DID MY EATING CHOICES IMPACT MY DAY?

Day 47: **Favorite Resources**

Product: HealthyOut Healthy Meal Finder (iOS & Android).
Cost: Free.
Note: We're not affiliated with this product - it's just a great tool.

The HealthyOut Healthy Meal Finder app will literally find healthy restaurant and grocery store meals that fit the personal food preferences and guidelines that you define. It can conform to specific mainstream diets, macronutrient ratios and even filters by cuisine and specific dishes. Their most popular filter: "Not a salad."

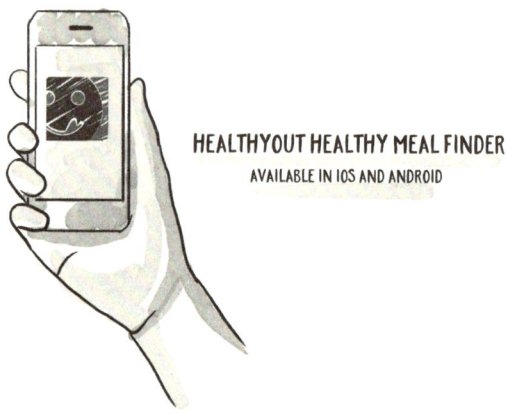

HEALTHYOUT HEALTHY MEAL FINDER
AVAILABLE IN IOS AND ANDROID

"Don't underestimate the power of thoughts and words. What you tell yourself every morning will set your mind and life on success." - Nina Bolivares

TODAY'S NUTRITION GOAL

DATE

_____ ☐

WATER DRINKING GOAL　　　　**EXERCISE GOAL**

_____ ☐　　_____ ☐

TODAY'S MEALS

Planned　　　　　　　Actual　　　　　Calories　　Protein / Carbs / Fat

SNACKS, DRINKS, & OTHER

TODAY'S TOTALS: _____ _____ _____ _____

HOW DID MY EATING CHOICES IMPACT MY DAY?

_____
_____
_____
_____

Day 48 : Favorite Podcasts

iTunes Reviews: 588

Podcast: *Ultimate Health* Podcast ★★★★⯪ 4.5
Hosts: Dr. Jesse Chappus & Marni Wasserman

Chappus retired from practicing as a chiropractor so that he could reach a much wider audience with his health message, and Wasserman is a nutritionist and chef. Both of these experts attribute their knowledge to their life experiences.

These two podcast superstars interview experts to answer pressing questions relating to physical, mental, and emotional wellness.

Check out their podcast on *iTunes*, *iHeart Radio*, *Stitcher*, or *Spreaker*. To find it you can simply search "Ultimate Health Podcast".

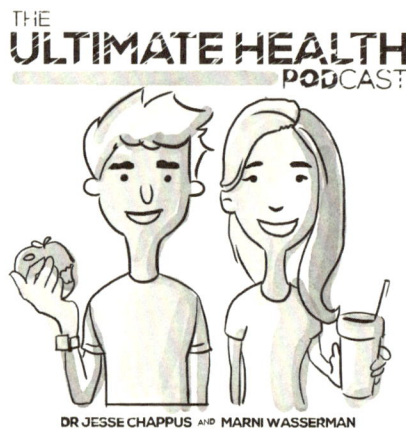

"Remember that when your body is hungry it wants NUTRIENTS, not calories." -Anonymous

TODAY'S NUTRITION GOAL

DATE

_____ ☐

💧 **WATER DRINKING GOAL**   🚶 **EXERCISE GOAL**

_____ ☐   _____ ☐

🍽 **TODAY'S MEALS**

📅 Planned	✓ Actual	Calories	Protein / Carbs / Fat

🍎 SNACKS, DRINKS, & OTHER

_____

_____

TODAY'S TOTALS: _____ _____ _____ _____

HOW DID MY EATING CHOICES IMPACT MY DAY?

_____

_____

_____

_____

Day 49: **Daily Challenge**

Challenge: Try carb cycling.

Here's the idea: You alternate between high-carb and low-carb days. The way it works, in theory, is that on high carb days, your body is able to restore glycogen stores to proper levels, and a rise in insulin helps the body avoid turning to muscle as a source of energy. On low-carb days you're maximizing fat burning.

Like any other piece of nutrition content, it doesn't apply equally to everybody. But Ari, one of the Habit Nest founders, is a huge proponent of carb cycling.

What to do:
1. On low-carb days, try to have 0.3 - 0.5 grams of carbohydrates per pound of body weight. On high-carb days, try to have 2 - 2.5 grams. Play around with these numbers depending on how much you exercise you get.
2. Start on a 5-day cycle during which you have three low-carb days, followed by two high-carb days.

**Note:* That doesn't mean eat a bunch of unhealthy carbs on high-carb days! Try to fill your quota with complex carbs.

☐ I completed this daily challenge.

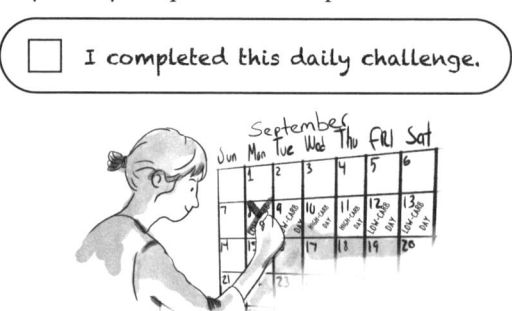

"Let food be thy medicine and medicine be thy food."
- Hippocrates

TODAY'S NUTRITION GOAL   DATE

_____ ☐

⬡ **WATER DRINKING GOAL**   🚶 **EXERCISE GOAL**

_____ ☐   _____ ☐

TODAY'S MEALS

| Planned | Actual | Calories | Protein / Carbs / Fat |

SNACKS, DRINKS, & OTHER

TODAY'S TOTALS: _____   _____ _____ _____

HOW DID MY EATING CHOICES IMPACT MY DAY?

_____
_____
_____
_____

Day 50: **Pro-Tip**

Learning to listen to your body.

If we began to speak the language of our body, we'd simultaneously appreciate it more *and* treat it better. For example, when our stomach is in pain or we're having difficulty going to the bathroom, our body is very seriously communicating information it wants us to act on. See if you can begin to better act on what your body communicates in the form of pain, feeing over-full, lethargic, etc.

Cut calories wherever you can.

In the end of the day, the less calories we consume, the better it is for our weight loss goals (up to a limit of course). A lot of the time we just don't realize how many extra calories we're eating when we take that extra handful of nuts, add that tablespoon of oil, use a lot of sauce, put a pack of butter on every piece of toast, etc.

Stay mindful of the excess calories you consume and try to see which corners you can begin to make a practice of cutting. They will add up quickly if you're consistent about it!

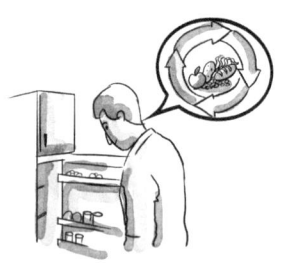

"To keep the body in good health is a duty, otherwise we shall not be able to keep our mind strong and clear."
-Buddha

TODAY'S NUTRITION GOAL

DATE

WATER DRINKING GOAL   **EXERCISE GOAL**

TODAY'S MEALS

Planned   Actual   Calories   Protein / Carbs / Fat

SNACKS, DRINKS, & OTHER

TODAY'S TOTALS: _____

HOW DID MY EATING CHOICES IMPACT MY DAY?

Day 51: **Daily Challenge**
Envision a realistic path for your eating habits a year from now.

Chances are, you know in your heart that in the long-term that your life would only be better if you found a healthy eating practice you stuck to. Make a shift from thinking short-term (even 66 days is tiny) to thinking of a clear, ambitious, long-term eating goal that you slowly move towards with experimentation over time.

You are now at least 51 days into this journey, if not many, many more (which is 100% okay). Take a good look at where you are now and where you started from.

Regardless of what the metric changes are in terms of shifts in body weight, take a look at all the small insights you've picked up along the way. That learning process is incredibly valuable.

It can be easy to set short-term sights for our nutrition goals, but that can often lead to a lot of self-sabotage and yo-yo dieting. Alternatively, we invite you to experiment with a longer-term view. What if you gave yourself 1-2 years to start reaching your dieting goals instead of 1-2 months? What if you made it your goal to learn as much as possible and passionately experiment, while being completely open to failing along the way?

This mental shift can help bring about a new approach to eating habits - one that invites constant learning of your body's relationship with food, rather than one of strict timelines, guilt, and pressure.

☐ I completed this daily challenge.

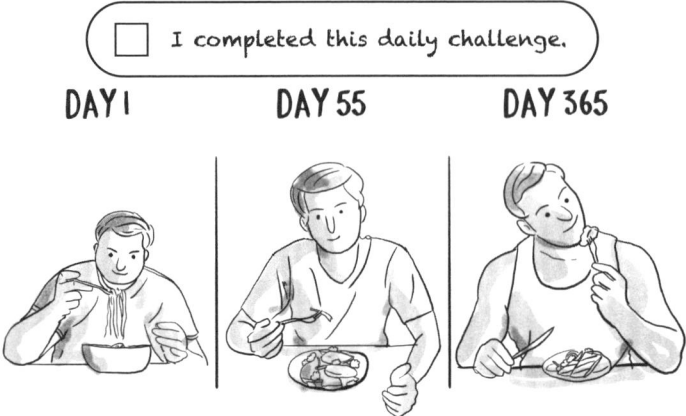

TODAY'S NUTRITION GOAL

DATE

_____ ☐

💧 **WATER DRINKING GOAL**   🚶 **EXERCISE GOAL**

_____ ☐   _____ ☐

🍴 **TODAY'S MEALS**

| 📅 Planned | ✓ Actual | Calories | Protein / Carbs / Fat |

🍎 SNACKS, DRINKS, & OTHER

TODAY'S TOTALS: _____   ____ ____ ____

HOW DID MY EATING CHOICES IMPACT MY DAY?

_____
_____
_____
_____

Day 52: **Affirmations**

1. Find a quiet area where you can do this in private so you can do this at ease. If you can't find a private space, say these in your head while pretending you're screaming them from a mountaintop.

2. Think of a time where you felt absolutely powerful - **where you felt on top of the world**. Tap into every emotion you had at that moment and get yourself into that state right now. How were you feeling then - Powerful? Unstoppable? Strong? Incredible!? Get into it now!!!!

3. Now feel your intensity grow tenfold! Say this with deep passion:

I live healthfully for myself, but also for those that I love so they may be empowered to improve their health as well. I enjoy being in my body and I nourish it every day. I do not take my body for granted.

Repeat this **one more time.**

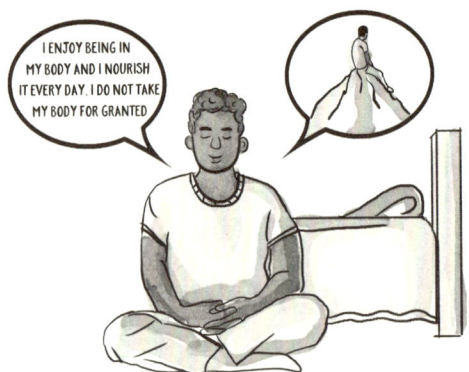

"The way I define happiness is being the creator of your experience, choosing to take pleasure in what you have, right now, regardless of the circumstances, while being the best you that you can be."
- Leo Babauta

⊕ TODAY'S NUTRITION GOAL

DATE

_____ ☐

◌ WATER DRINKING GOAL   🚶 EXERCISE GOAL

_____ ☐   _____ ☐

🍽 TODAY'S MEALS

📅 Planned	✓ Actual	Calories	Protein / Carbs / Fat

🍎 SNACKS, DRINKS, & OTHER

_____

_____

TODAY'S TOTALS: _____ ___ ___ ___

HOW DID MY EATING CHOICES IMPACT MY DAY?

_____

_____

_____

Day 53: **Daily Challenge**

You do not have to listen to your cravings.

Although cravings lessen in strength and quantity over time, making the right food choices never becomes completely mindless. The key is to remember that your cravings don't have to be listened to. Successful healthy eaters feel cravings just like anyone else, they just learn not to pay attention to them.

By refusing to give into a craving, you are literally taking power from it. A craving is just a passing thought like any other unless you give it the power to control your action. You are your ACTIONS, not your passing thoughts.

In summary:
- Your mindset changes from your actions.
- You always have control over your actions (while you can't control the thoughts that come through your head).

So… take the right actions to succeed, regardless of your emotional state. You emotions will be set by the actions you take.

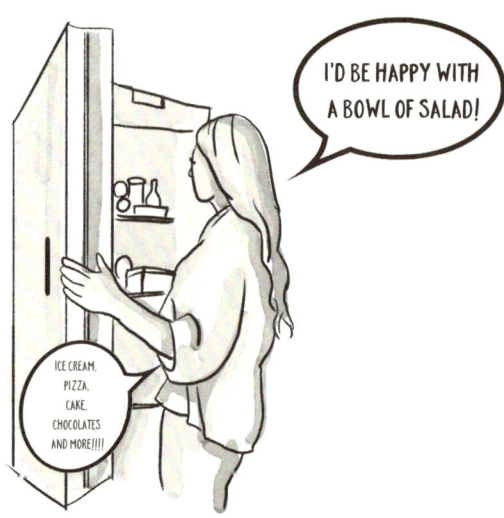

○ **TODAY'S NUTRITION GOAL** DATE

_____ ☐

💧 **WATER DRINKING GOAL**   🚶 **EXERCISE GOAL**

_____ ☐   _____ ☐

🍽 **TODAY'S MEALS**

📅 Planned   ✓ Actual   Calories   Protein / Carbs / Fat

🍎 SNACKS, DRINKS, & OTHER

TODAY'S TOTALS: _____

HOW DID MY EATING CHOICES IMPACT MY DAY?

Day 54: **Pro-Tip**

The most bang for your buck.

A study on cardiovascular exercise was conducted in which ten men and ten women were split into two groups. One group ran for thirty-to-sixty minutes on a treadmill three times a week, while the other group did four-to-six 30-second sprints three times per week.

Think about the difference, 90 - 180 minutes a week vs. 6-9 minutes.

In the group who ran for 30-60 minutes a week, fat mass decreased by an average of 5.8%, but in the group who ran sprints fat mass decreased by 12.4%!

This is the only page in this journal that deals with exercise over the specifics of nutrition but we wanted to emphasize it because it's important as hell. High intensity interval training works and if your goal is to burn fat and save time and energy, there is no better option.

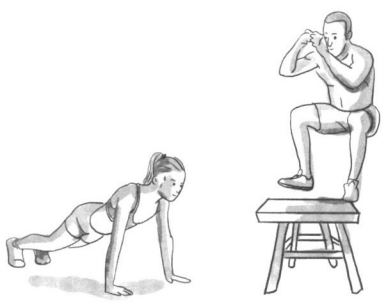

"Don't underestimate the power of thoughts and words. What you tell yourself every morning will set your mind and life on that path. Talk success, victory, happiness and blessings over your destiny."
– Nina Bolivare

TODAY'S NUTRITION GOAL

DATE

WATER DRINKING GOAL

EXERCISE GOAL

TODAY'S MEALS

Planned | Actual | Calories | Protein / Carbs / Fat

SNACKS, DRINKS, & OTHER

TODAY'S TOTALS: _____

HOW DID MY EATING CHOICES IMPACT MY DAY?

Day 55: **Success Story**

Kesha. Writer, musician, struggled with an eating disorder.

In 2014, Kesha checked herself into an undisclosed rehab facility to receive treatment for an eating disorder.

She emerged stronger and with an empowering perspective that she shared with her fans: "I felt like a liar, telling people to love themselves as they are, while I was being hateful to myself and really hurting my body. I wanted to control things that weren't in my power, but I was controlling the wrong things. I convinced myself that being sick, being skinny was part of my job."

Kesha focuses on not giving in to what others think about her body and realizing that eating is actually healthy.

A healthy relationship with food is an extremely important aspect of each of our lives. That requires eating.

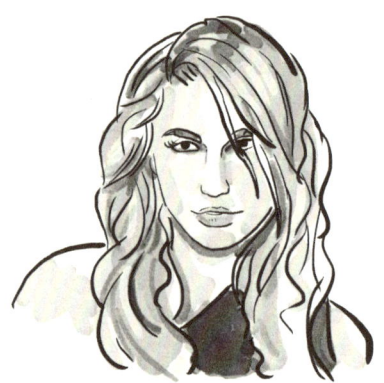

"I have always been delighted at the prospect of a new day, a fresh try, one more start, with perhaps a bit of magic waiting somewhere behind the morning." - B. Priestley

TODAY'S NUTRITION GOAL DATE

_____ ☐

💧 **WATER DRINKING GOAL**   🚶 **EXERCISE GOAL**

_____ ☐   _____ ☐

🍽 **TODAY'S MEALS**

📅 Planned   ✓ Actual   Calories   Protein / Carbs / Fat

🍎 SNACKS, DRINKS, & OTHER

TODAY'S TOTALS: _____

HOW DID MY EATING CHOICES IMPACT MY DAY?

Day 56: Affirmations

4. Find a quiet area where you can do this in private so you can do this at ease. If you can't find a private space, say these in your head while pretending you're screaming them from a mountaintop.

5. Think of a time where you felt absolutely powerful - **where you felt on top of the world**. Tap into every emotion you had at that moment and get yourself into that state right now. How were you feeling then - Powerful? Unstoppable? Strong? Incredible!? Get into it now!!!!

6. Now feel your intensity grow tenfold! Say this with deep passion:

My body is my temple. Everything I bring into my temple belongs there and serves a purpose. I no longer ONLY eat based on taste. I am in control of my appetite and thus, in control of my food choices.

Repeat this **one more time**.

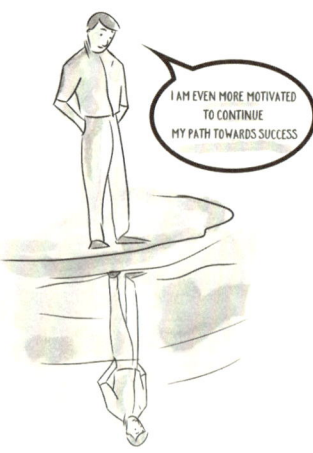

"If you don't take care of your body, where are you going to live?"
- Unknown

TODAY'S NUTRITION GOAL

DATE

WATER DRINKING GOAL

EXERCISE GOAL

TODAY'S MEALS

Planned | Actual | Calories | Protein / Carbs / Fat

SNACKS, DRINKS, & OTHER

TODAY'S TOTALS: ____

HOW DID MY EATING CHOICES IMPACT MY DAY?

Progress Tracker (Optional)

Progress Picture (Front)

Progress Picture (Side)

How happy am I with myself (circle one)?

1   2   3   4   5

_____   _____
Previous Weight   Previous Body Fat %

_____   _____
Weight   Body Fat %

Day 57: **Pro-Tip**

<u>*Test removing foods for 1-2 weeks.*</u>

In order to find out how YOUR body is affected by different types of foods and strategies, you have to experiment a lot and give these experiments time to give you the information you need.

You also have to be very thorough so you know exactly what change is causing the corresponding reaction you see. If you make too many changes to your diet at once, you won't know which change to attribute your body's reaction to.

1. Make 1-2 changes consistently for a week or two at a time.
2. Pay close attention to how your energy levels, mood, and appearance are affected.

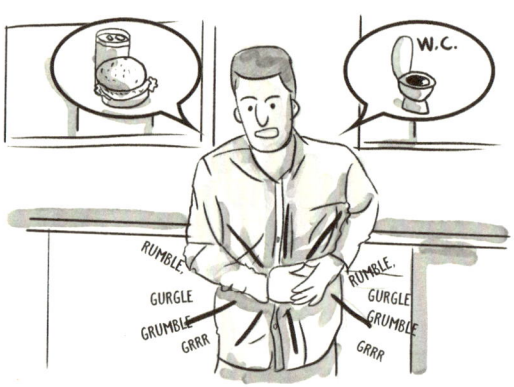

"The spirit cannot endure the body when overfed, but, if underfed, the body cannot endure the spirit."
- St. Frances de Sales

TODAY'S NUTRITION GOAL   DATE
_____   ☐

WATER DRINKING GOAL   **EXERCISE GOAL**
_____ ☐   _____ ☐

TODAY'S MEALS

Planned	Actual	Calories	Protein / Carbs / Fat

SNACKS, DRINKS, & OTHER

_____

TODAY'S TOTALS: _____

HOW DID MY EATING CHOICES IMPACT MY DAY?

_____
_____
_____
_____

Day 58: **YouTube Alert!**

462,000+ SUBSCRIBERS

Fit Men Cook.

This is an AWESOME channel. When the host Kevin Curry wanted to get in shape, he realized after some time that he could not out-train his diet. He realized he would never have the body he wanted without eating the right foods.

After experimenting on his own with healthy, cheap and tasty meals, he made a YouTube channel that has grown to be sensational. He shares videos about shopping for the right foods, with specific, easy-to-make recipes and meal preps.

Subscribe for free here: **https://www.youtube.com/user/fitmencook/**

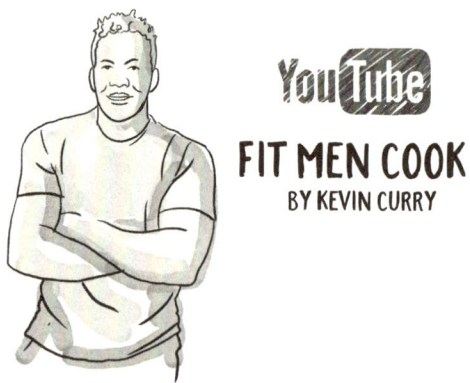

"Tell me what you eat and I will tell you who you are."
- Brillat-Savarin

⊕ **TODAY'S NUTRITION GOAL** DATE

_____ ☐

◌ **WATER DRINKING GOAL**   🚶 **EXERCISE GOAL**

_____ ☐   _____ ☐

🍴 **TODAY'S MEALS**

📅 Planned	✓ Actual	Calories	Protein / Carbs / Fat

🍎 SNACKS, DRINKS, & OTHER

_____

_____

TODAY'S TOTALS: _____ ____ ____ ____

HOW DID MY EATING CHOICES IMPACT MY DAY?

_____

_____

_____

_____

Day 59: Success Story

Jonah Hill. Actor, producer, screenwriter & comedian; Lost 40 pounds.

If you remember what Jonah Hill looked like in his first big movie - *Superbad* - you'll remember he was extremely overweight. If you check out how he looks now, you'll be completely shocked. He's just your average skinny guy!

On the Jimmy Fallon show, Hill said, "I gained weight for this movie *War Dogs*, and then I wanted to get in better shape, so I called Channing Tatum, and said, 'Hey, if I eat less and go to a trainer, will I get in better shape?' And he said, 'Yes, [of course you will], it's the simplest thing in the entire world.'"

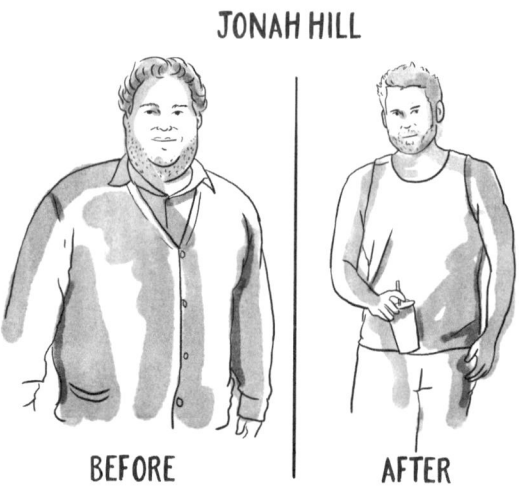

"At the most elite level, your nutrition becomes a lifestyle- you just do it."
-Abby Wambach

TODAY'S NUTRITION GOAL

DATE

_____ ☐

WATER DRINKING GOAL **EXERCISE GOAL**

_____ ☐ _____ ☐

TODAY'S MEALS

Planned   Actual   Calories   Protein / Carbs / Fat

SNACKS, DRINKS, & OTHER

TODAY'S TOTALS: _____

HOW DID MY EATING CHOICES IMPACT MY DAY?

Day 60: Pro-Tip

Ready to work towards a new habit goal!?

If you've gotten this far, you've had a strong taste for how much eating healthier and having a sense of control over your weight impacts your overall quality of life.

It's the perfect time to begin thinking about how other success habits can also improve your day to day experience of life in beautiful ways.

If you're ready to work on other habits, you can check out:

1. The *Morning Sidekick Journal*: habitnest.com/mornings
2. The *Meditation Sidekick Journal*: habitnest.com/meditation
3. The *Badass Body Goals Fitness Journal*: habitnest.com/badass
4. The *Weightlifting Gym Buddy Journal*: habitnest.com/weightlifting

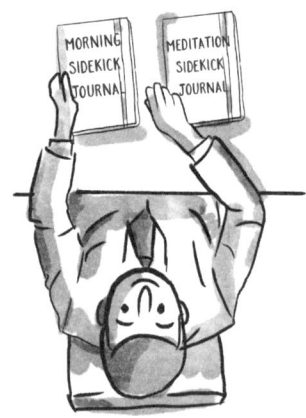

"It is well to be up before daybreak, for such habits contribute to health, wealth, and wisdom." - Aristotle

TODAY'S NUTRITION GOAL DATE _____

_____ ☐

WATER DRINKING GOAL   **EXERCISE GOAL**

_____ ☐   _____ ☐

TODAY'S MEALS

Planned	Actual	Calories	Protein / Carbs / Fat
_____	_____	_____	_____
_____	_____	_____	_____
_____	_____	_____	_____
....	....	....	....
....	....	....	....

SNACKS, DRINKS, & OTHER

_____ _____ _____

_____ _____ _____

TODAY'S TOTALS: _____ _____

HOW DID MY EATING CHOICES IMPACT MY DAY?

_____

_____

_____

_____

Day 61: **Daily Challenge**

Challenge: Get someone else on the healthy eating wagon!

One way to hold yourself accountable to making a positive change is by having a partner alongside you.

But the ULTIMATE form of accountability is seeing success in yourself, which, in turn, encourages others to adopt the same positive behavior. When you preach, you have basically no choice to practice. You're on Day 56 of this journal - regardless of how close or far you are from your ultimate goal, you've come an insanely long way towards incorporating healthier eating into your daily routine.

Choose a friend or loved one who you know needs the inspiration and knowledge you've gained. Motivate them through your own story and help them understand that they CAN change their eating habits with slow and consistent effort.

You have the power to change other people's lives, which will motivate you to continue on your own path of change.

☐ I completed this daily challenge.

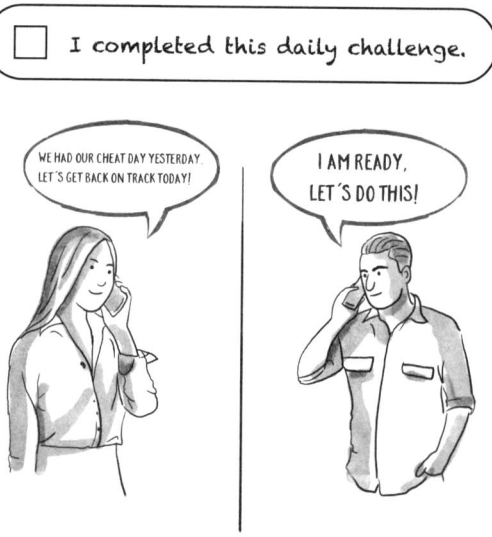

TODAY'S NUTRITION GOAL   DATE

_____ ☐

WATER DRINKING GOAL   **EXERCISE GOAL**

_____ ☐   _____ ☐

TODAY'S MEALS

Planned   Actual   Calories   Protein / Carbs / Fat

SNACKS, DRINKS, & OTHER

TODAY'S TOTALS: _____   ____ ____ ____

HOW DID MY EATING CHOICES IMPACT MY DAY?

Day 62: **Pro-Tip**

Make your cravings work FOR you.

When it comes to cravings we usually start out by hating ourselves for being tempted, doing all that we can to resist the craving, ultimately giving up and then feeling extremely guilty about it. Feeling guilty about it causes us to feel like failures which tends to lead to failing again rather than push us in the direction we want to move.

One way to avoid feeling guilty about giving in to temptation (which we all do) is to condition it on the success of a mini-goal. For example, promise yourself that you'll only eat that donut or cookie you're craving if you follow through on your lunch plan. That way, you avoid feeling bad about it and it doesn't snowball into repeated 'failure.'

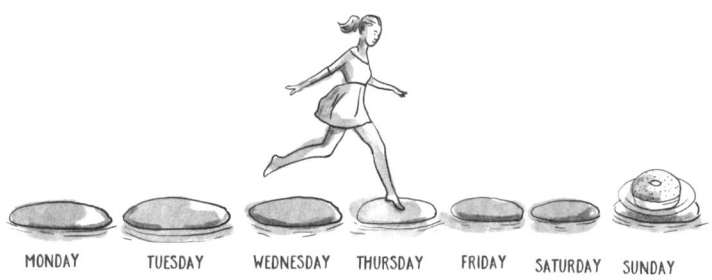

"Imagine how much easier life would be if we were born with a user guide or owner's manual to could tell us what to eat & how to live healthy."
-Erika M. Szabo

TODAY'S NUTRITION GOAL　　　　　　　DATE

_____ ☐

WATER DRINKING GOAL　　　　**EXERCISE GOAL**

_____ ☐　　_____ ☐

TODAY'S MEALS

Planned　　　　　Actual　　　　Calories　　Protein / Carbs / Fat

SNACKS, DRINKS, & OTHER

TODAY'S TOTALS: _____　____　____　____

HOW DID MY EATING CHOICES IMPACT MY DAY?

Day 63: **Affirmations**

1. Find a quiet area where you can do this in private so you can do this at ease. If you can't find a private space, say these in your head while pretending you're screaming them from a mountaintop.

2. Think of a time where you felt absolutely powerful - **where you felt on top of the world**. Tap into every emotion you had at that moment and get yourself into that state right now. How were you feeling then - Powerful? Unstoppable? Strong? Incredible!? Get into it now!!!!

3. Now feel your intensity grow tenfold! Say this with deep passion:

*Day after day, I am realizing that my potential in life is **absolutely limitless**. I am an unstoppable force for good.*

I am going to destroy every obstacle and challenge that comes in my path because I know that nothing is bigger than me.

By improving myself every day, day after day after day, I am creating a snowball effect that will propel me through life to incredible success.

Repeat this **one more time.**

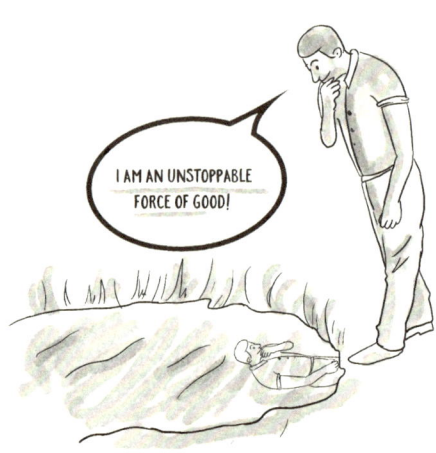

TODAY'S NUTRITION GOAL ☐ DATE _____

_____

💧 **WATER DRINKING GOAL** ☐   🚶 **EXERCISE GOAL** ☐

_____   _____

🍽 **TODAY'S MEALS**

Planned	Actual	Calories	Protein / Carbs / Fat

🍎 SNACKS, DRINKS, & OTHER

TODAY'S TOTALS: _____

HOW DID MY EATING CHOICES IMPACT MY DAY?

_____
_____
_____
_____

Day 64: **Pro-Tip**

The next time you feel 'out of it,' take physical action (not mental) to shift your body's state.

Preparing for your off days and days of struggle is absolutely critical. It's what many of the Pro-Tips in this book cover. Shifting your off days to work in your favor is what's most challenging, yet the most rewarding.

Let's be real - having an off day is inevitable and you will absolutely hit another point where you feel like total crap. Trying to mentally battle yourself to "feel better" won't do you any good in this state.

What IS incredibly effective is taking a **physical action** to shock your body physiologically. The next time you feel out of it, force yourself to take a physical action to shift your body's state (by boosting oxygen, adrenaline, and/or endorphins). Some specific actions you can take the next time you feel out of it are:

1. Take 5 long inhales deep into your stomach.
2. Work out or move around (even for 30 seconds).
3. Take a cold shower (this is for the truly crazy ones out there).

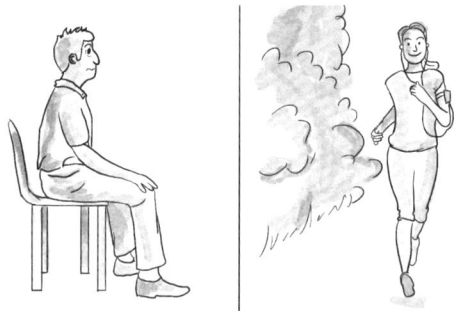

"Health is like money. We never have a true idea of its value until we lose it." - Josh Billings

TODAY'S NUTRITION GOAL

DATE

_____ ☐

WATER DRINKING GOAL

EXERCISE GOAL

_____ ☐   _____ ☐

TODAY'S MEALS

Planned	Actual	Calories	Protein / Carbs / Fat

SNACKS, DRINKS, & OTHER

TODAY'S TOTALS: _____   ____ ____ ____

HOW DID MY EATING CHOICES IMPACT MY DAY?

_____
_____
_____
_____

Day 65: Success Story

John Goodman. Actor; Lost 100+ lbs

On past weight loss:

"I used to go on these diets, take three months and lose about 60-70 pounds, feel great, and reward myself with crapola. Twinkies look good."

On his current transformation:

"I took it slow. I just wanted to change my lifestyle. You look in the mirror everyday and go, 'I gotta deal with this the rest of the day, I gotta deal with this schmuck?'"

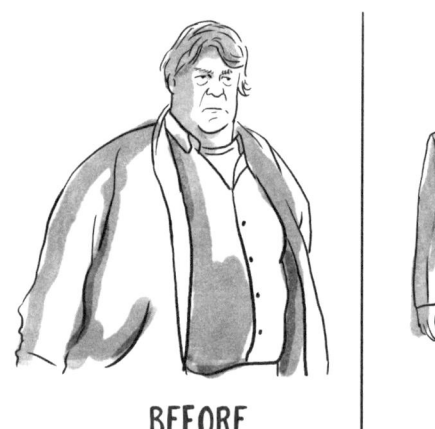

"Our bodies are our gardens – our wills are our gardeners."
- William Shakespeare

TODAY'S NUTRITION GOAL DATE

WATER DRINKING GOAL   **EXERCISE GOAL**

TODAY'S MEALS

Planned	Actual	Calories	Protein / Carbs / Fat

SNACKS, DRINKS, & OTHER

TODAY'S TOTALS: _____

HOW DID MY EATING CHOICES IMPACT MY DAY?

Day 66: Congratulations!!!

You've made it to the end of the journal. **You have now transformed your eating habits,** one of the most difficult habits to master.

For you to have gotten this far means you've earned a very serious congratulations. You need to celebrate because your willpower and confidence should be soaring through the roof. You've learned lessons about yourself not many dare to approach. You've struggled with your own mind, body and heart and gained some serious control over them. You fully understand that you have the power in you to accomplish ANY goal you put your mind to.

This is a skill you've built inside you that you can turn on whenever you need it at any future point in your lifetime. **That's so awesome.**

You are a WARRIOR and us three (Amir, Ari, & Mikey) hope you continue to build on your habit success and personal development for the rest of your life.

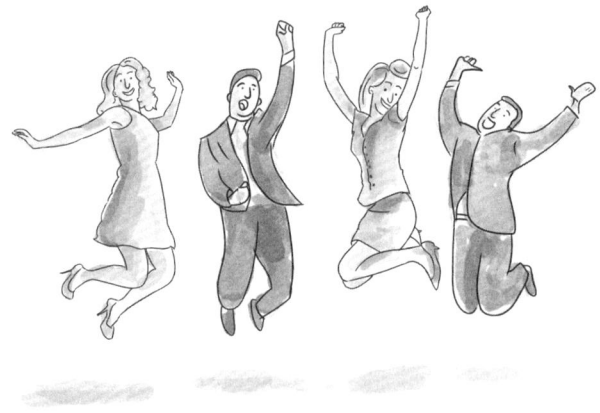

TODAY'S NUTRITION GOAL　　　　　　　DATE

_____   ☐

◌ **WATER DRINKING GOAL**　　　🚶 **EXERCISE GOAL**

_____ ☐　　_____ ☐

TODAY'S MEALS

Planned	Actual	Calories	Protein / Carbs / Fat
_____	_____	_____	_____
_____	_____	_____	_____
_____	_____	_____	_____
....	....	....	....
....	....	....	....

🍎 SNACKS, DRINKS, & OTHER

_____

_____

TODAY'S TOTALS: _____ ___ ___ ___

HOW DID MY EATING CHOICES IMPACT MY DAY?

_____

_____

_____

_____

PHASE 3. COMPLETED.

Phase 3 Recap: Days 22-66+

1. Think about what your life looked like before you began this habit - what are you doing differently now? How do you feel?

___

2. What unforeseen effects has your life gained from all this?

___

3. When you are struggling with this habit in the future, what are the key factors you should remember to do again?

___

4. What daily tracking & accountability can you have going forward to maintain the momentum you've built here?

___

Progress Tracker (Optional)

Progress Picture
(Front)

Progress Picture
(Side)

How happy am I with myself (circle one)?

1   2   3   4   5

_____   _____
Previous Weight   Previous Body Fat %

_____   _____
Weight   Body Fat %

- Fin -

So... What Now?

Although you should feel very accomplished for getting through this entire journal... know that you built this habit to *continually improve your life. Don't stop now. This is only the beginning.*

One huge factor to this is tracking your progress. Once you stop tracking, it makes it exponentially easier for you to stop paying attention to your food intake (due to the lack of accountability with yourself).

Remember: **Every single day in your life where you plan your meals with focus and intent will automatically be a better day of your life.**

You only stand to gain from continuing this habit.

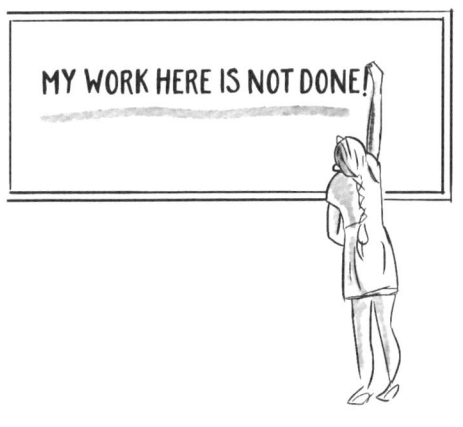

What Life-Changing Habit Will YOU Conquer Next?

Did you enjoy your *Nutrition Sidekick Journal*? We poured our hearts and souls into it so we're glad.

Here are some other products from our team that were built with all the love in the world to be truly effective at impacting people's lives.

Meet The Habit Nest Team

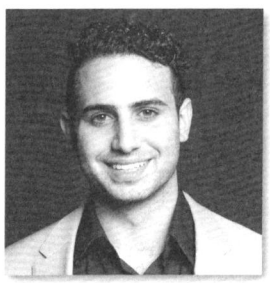

Amir Atighehchi graduated from USC's Marshall School of Business in 2013. He got his first taste of entrepreneurship during college with Mikey when they co-founded a bicycle lock company called *Nutlock*. It wasn't until after college when he opened his eyes to the world of personal development and healthy habits. Amir is fascinated by creative challenges and entrepreneurship.

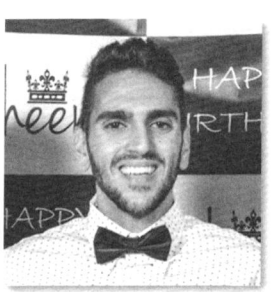

Mikey Ahdoot transformed his life from a 200+ pound, video game addict to someone who was doing 17 daily habits consistently at one point. From ice cold showers to brainstorming 10 ideas a day (shoutout to James Altucher) to celebrating life every single day, he first hand is becoming a habit routine machine that sets himself up for success daily. He is a graduate of USC's Marshall School of Business and a proud Trojan.

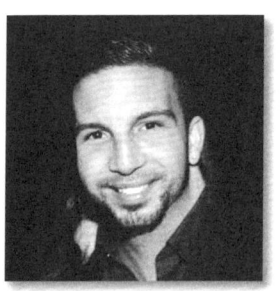

Ari Banayan graduated from the University of Southern California Gould School of Law in 2016. Through his own life experience, he understands how important it is to take care of ourselves mentally, physically and emotionally to operate at maximum capacity. He uses waking up early, reading, meditation, exercise, and a healthy diet to create a solid foundation for his everyday life.

Read all of our full stories here:
habitnest.com/aboutus

Shop Habit Nest Products

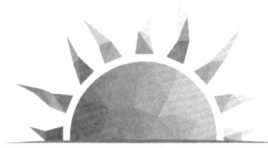

Morning Sidekick
Journal

The Morning Sidekick Journal is the first journal we created at Habit Nest. It has a similar layout as the *Nutrition Sidekick Journal,* consisting of 66 days of content and 66 days of tracking.

Morning routines are shown to be one of the most **critical elements of winning your day.** Starting your day off on the right foot sets the tone for the rest of it.

The journal is specifically designed to **create a cycle of accountability** within yourself by using your nights to hold you accountable in the morning, and your mornings to map out what's needed for that night.

It's jam-packed with effective and actionable content that will help you build this habit in bite sized chunks.

Like all of our products, the *Morning Sidekick Journal* comes with a 50-year satisfaction guarantee.

One thing we love: Regardless of what time you wake up, the journal will show you how to create a routine (short or long) that works for you.

Get yours at **habitnest.com/morning**

Sample Journal Page

DATE _____

🌙 TONIGHT I'LL SLEEP AT: __11:30pm__ & TOMORROW I'LL WAKE UP AT: __6:30am__

Night 0
(Begin Nighttime Routine.)

✨ **MEMORABLE MOMENT(S) I EXPERIENCED TODAY:**

Watching the sunrise on my morning run :)

Finally made progress on my side-business!

☀️ **MY MORNING RITUAL TOMORROW WILL BE:**   *Completed?*

1. 5 minutes of meditation ✓
2. Read 2 pages of "Think and Grow Rich" ✓
3. Affirmations ☐
4. Walk 2 blocks outside ☐
5. Plan out and strategize the rest of my day ☐

☀️ LAST NIGHT I SLEPT AT: __12am__ & WOKE UP TODAY AT: __7am__

Day 1
(Begin Morning Routine.)

🐎 **MY MOST IMPORTANT TASK FOR TODAY IS:**

Begin designing the app for my new startup

⏱ **ONE WAY I CAN IMPROVE LIFE BY 1% IS:**

Less Facebook / Instagram in the mornings

🧘 **TOP TWO DISTRACTIONS TO MINIMIZE TONIGHT (BEFORE BED):**

1. Watching YouTube in bed (limit: 15mins)
2. Watching the news (limit: 15mins)

Meditation Sidekick
Journal

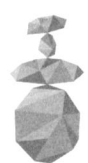

The *Meditation Sidekick Journal* is built to help two types of people:

1. To help **newcomers or past strugglers** easily own the practice of meditation.

2. To help **constant meditators** push their practice to another level.

Layout of the journal

1. **Building the foundation** - get a quick insight into the *science behind meditation* and get an idea of what you're likely to experience during it.

2. **Accountability** - track your practice daily to see your progress and hold yourself accountable in staying consistent.

3. **Learn in bite-sized chunks** - get daily exposure to different types of meditations (e.g. transcendental, gratitude, physical body, etc.) and see which ones impact your life the most.

One thing we love: The journal is not just designed to help you meditate effectively, but more importantly, to **help you reach the end goal of consistently living mindfully every day.**

Get yours at habitnest.com/meditation

Sample Journal Page

DATE

 TODAY I WILL MEDITATE AT: **FOR AT LEAST:**

7:30 a.m. ✓   5 minutes ✓

ONE UPCOMING MENTAL OR EMOTIONAL HURDLE TO BE MINDFUL OF:

My presentation for my boss at work — own it!

BENEFITS I FELT TODAY (CIRCLE):

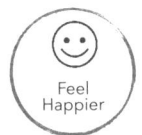 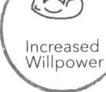  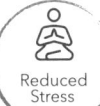

Feel Happier | More Creative | Increased Willpower | Improved Focus | More Energized | Reduced Stress

 WHAT DOES MY INTERNAL DIALOGUE CONSIST OF?

I realize that I think about my appearance A LOT... and I immediately assume people judge me for it.

 ONE SMALL WAY I CAN IMPROVE MY INTERNAL DIALOGUE:

I could be more understanding when I'm feeling self-conscious and willingly accept myself for how I look.

OPENING UP ABOUT MY DAY:

Today was a rollercoaster. I realize that when I'm working with others, I prefer not to rely on them to get things done. It's something I want to work on improving because I make myself feel anxious when it happens.

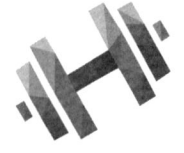

The Weightlifting Gym Buddy
Journal

The Weightlifting Gym Buddy Journal is a complete 12-week personal training program.

No thinking required, just open the journal, follow the workouts, and track your progress. The journal is designed to accompany you to the gym, to help you track your weight/reps for each workout, and to help you compete against yourself every workout.

- Contains 60 guided workouts for you to follow

- Each day's workout targets 2 muscle groups

- For lifters of all levels to push themselves to the next level and maximize competition with themselves

- Each workout takes 45-60 minutes

- Number of reps to aim for is already set for you

- Built with a pyramid weight/rep format to intensify each exercise dramatically

- No thinking required - just open the journal and follow along for amazing results

- Alternative exercises are listed in the case your gym is missing a specific machine

Get yours at habitnest.com/weightlifting

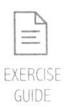 (You'll see links to exercise guides here each day)
EXERCISE GUIDE

Sample Workout: Biceps & Triceps

DATE _____

1. PREACHER CURL
(ALTERNATIVE: SEATED DUMBBELL CURL)

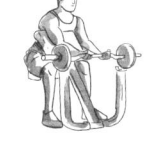 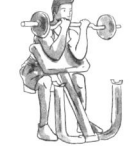

PREVIOUS BEST   REPS: __5__   WEIGHT: __60__

SET 1   REPS: __14__   (GOAL: 10-15)   WEIGHT: __40__

SET 2   REPS: __10__   (GOAL: 8-12)   WEIGHT: __50__

SET 3   REPS: __7__   (GOAL: 6-8)   WEIGHT: __60__

SET 4   REPS: __6__   (GOAL: 4-6)   WEIGHT: __60__
(OPTIONAL)

2. CLOSE GRIP BENCH PRESS

(By having your "Previous Best" reps and weight values listed for each specific exercise, you'll have a clear target to beat weekly.)

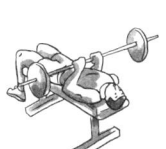 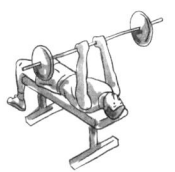 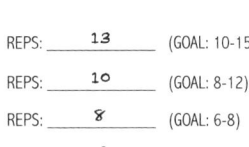

PREVIOUS BEST   REPS: __5__   WEIGHT: __50__

SET 1   REPS: __13__   (GOAL: 10-15)   WEIGHT: __30__

SET 2   REPS: __10__   (GOAL: 8-12)   WEIGHT: __40__

SET 3   REPS: __8__   (GOAL: 6-8)   WEIGHT: __50__

SET 4   REPS: __5__   (GOAL: 4-6)   WEIGHT: __50__
(OPTIONAL)

3. ROPE HAMMER CURL

(The fourth set on each exercise is optional but highly recommended.)

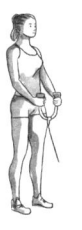 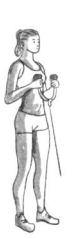

PREVIOUS BEST   REPS: __6__   WEIGHT: __50__

SET 1   REPS: __11__   (GOAL: 10-15)   WEIGHT: __35__

SET 2   REPS: __11__   (GOAL: 8-12)   WEIGHT: __45__

SET 3   REPS: __7__   (GOAL: 6-8)   WEIGHT: __50__

SET 4   REPS: __–__   (GOAL: 4-6)   WEIGHT: __–__
(OPTIONAL)

4. OVERHEAD DUMBBELL EXTENSION

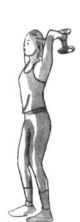 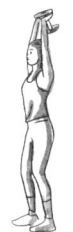

PREVIOUS BEST   REPS: __4__   WEIGHT: __55__

SET 1   REPS: __14__   (GOAL: 10-15)   WEIGHT: __35__

SET 2   REPS: __12__   (GOAL: 8-12)   WEIGHT: __45__

SET 3   REPS: __6__   (GOAL: 6-8)   WEIGHT: __45__

SET 4   REPS: __5__   (GOAL: 4-6)   WEIGHT: __55__
(OPTIONAL)

 TODAY'S WORKOUT INTENSITY: __8.5__ / 10

The Badass Body Goals Booty Shaping & Resistance Training
Journal

The Badass Body Goals Booty Shaping & Resistance Training Journal is a full 10-week personal training program which includes 50 guided workouts that are each unique, engaging, and challenging.

The journal is co-written by fitness expert Jennifer Cohen and has a large focus on circuit training (60% of the journal) with a variety of weight training for the remainder.

- The journal is designed to be done at home or in the gym with weights if you want to use more resistance.

- Every journal comes with a timed video guide that allows you to do the workout from beginning to end by simply following along each day.

- Track your results by filling in certain important variables as you complete each workout. As a result, you'll be getting constant encouragement by seeing first-hand how quickly you're improving.

- The journal contains an optimal mix of 4-3-2-1 interval circuits and resistance training workouts workout days. The two are designed to keep you engaged with different movements for short periods which will optimize fat loss and muscle development at the same time.

Get yours at **habitnest.com/badass**

EXERCISE GUIDE
https://HabitNest.link/booty01

Workout 1: 4-3-2-1

DATE _____

GLUTE ACTIVATION WARMUP
(30s EACH)

a. Clam Opener

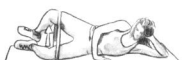
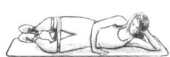

(30s Each Leg)

b. Glute Bridge w/ Band Flutter

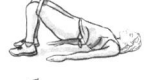
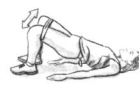

c. Fire Hydrant

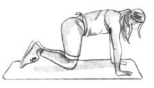
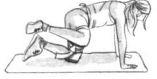

(30s Each Side)

d. Lateral Leg Raise

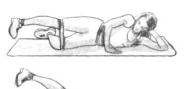
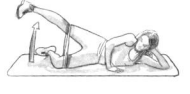

- 30s Each Leg (w/ Foot Flexed)
- 30s Each Leg (w/ Toes Pointing Down)

---------- 30 SECOND BREAK ----------

CIRCUIT 1
(60s EACH)

1a. Curtsy Lunge   **1b. Curtsy Lunge**   **1c. Boxing Jab**   **1d. Side to Side Squat**

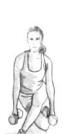 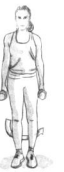 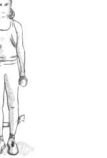 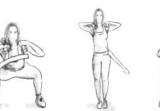

REPS: _____ → REPS: _____ → REPS: _____ → REPS: _____
(Left Leg)   (Right Leg)

---------- 30 SECOND BREAK ----------

CIRCUIT 2
(50s EACH)

2a. 180° Jump Twist to Floor Tap   **2b. Squat to Overhead Press**   **2c. Plie Jump Squat**

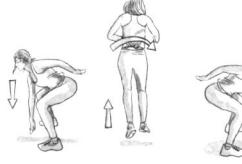 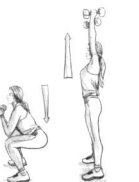 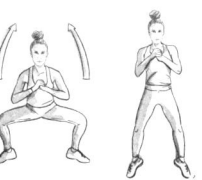

SET 1 REPS: _____ → SET 1 REPS: _____ → SET 1 REPS: _____

SET 2 REPS: _____ → SET 2 REPS: _____ → SET 2 REPS: _____

Share the Love

If you're reading this, that means you've come pretty far from where you were when starting. You should be extremely proud of yourself!

If you believe this journal has had a positive impact on your life, we invite you to consider gifting a new one to a friend.

Is there a holiday coming up? Is there a special birthday around the corner? Or do you just want to put a smile on someone's face and do something incredible for them?

Gifting this journal is the absolute best way to show any gratitude you may have for what we've written here, as well as serving as a force of good through giving back to others. And you can rest assured that you're helping improve another person's life at the same time.

We created a discount code for getting this far that can be used for any Nutrition Sidekick Journal reorder (make sure to use the same email address you placed the order with).

If you decide to, feel free to re-order here:
habitnest.com/nutrition

Use code **MeanLean15** for 15% off!

Content Index

Progress Tracker..Check-In #1

Day 1: Pro-Tip....................Set your food goals the night before

Day 2: Pro-Tip..........................Outsmart your hunger hormone

Day 3: Daily Challenge......Pay attention your daily mini-decisions

Day 4: Pro-Tip...............Applying the three principles of nutrition

Day 5: Pro-Tip……..Experiment with high-protein food alternatives

Day 6: Daily Challenge...............Try intermittent fasting for a day

Day 7: Pro-Tip...............It's better in the trash than your stomach

Day 8: Success Story..........Mikey Ahdoot, co-author of this journal

Day 9: Daily Challenge...............What factors have impeded you?

Day 10: Pro-Tip...…...............Drink naturally flavored water

Day 11: Affirmations......................................Affirmation #1

Day 12: Success Story.......................................Tony Robbins

Day 13: Pro-Tip...........................One cheat meal every 3 days

Day 14: Favorite Resources.........................*The Fooducate app.*

Progress Tracker..Check-In #2

Day 15: Double Daily Challenge............Juice + low-calorie snacks

Day 16: Affirmations..Affirmation #2

Day 17: Pro-Tip...................Make use of vitamins & supplements

Day 18: Daily Challenge...................Try meal prepping for a night

Day 19: YouTube Alert!................................*Clean & Delicious*

Day 20: Affirmations..Affirmation #3

Day 21: Daily Challenge..........Incorporate more resistance training

Day 22: Pro-Tip..Keep it simple

Day 23: Daily Challenge...Party smart

Day 24: Affirmations..Affirmation #4

Day 25: Super Read................*In Defense of Food by Michael Pollan*

Day 26: Daily Challenge...............The one-week gallon challenge

Day 27: Pro-Tip.....................................Do NOT do diet soda

Day 28: Affirmations..Affirmation #5

Progress Tracker...Check-In #3

Day 29: Favorite Podcasts........................*No Meat Athlete Radio*

Day 30: Pro-Tip................................Audit your calorie counting

Day 31: Affirmation...Affirmation #6

Day 32: Pro-Tip.........Creative ways to satisfy sweet tooth cravings

Day 33: Pro-Tip……………Maintaining can be more difficult than losing.

Day 34: Success Story………………………………….Zach Galifinakis

Day 35: Affirmations……………………..……………..….Affirmation #7

Day 36: Success Story…………………………..……...Melissa McCarthy

Day 37: Daily Challenge…………..Remove your images of perfection

Day 38: Favorite Resources………….*Accu-Measure* body fat caliper

Day 39: Pro-Tip……………………………….Your kitchen tells the future

Day 40: Daily Challenge…….Think about actions today vs. tomorrow

Day 41: Pro-Tip………………………………………………….Chew, a lot.

Day 42: Favorite Podcasts…………………….*The Sound Bites Podcast*

Progress Tracker……………………………………….Check-In #4

Day 43: Affirmations…………………………….……….Affirmation #8

Day 44: Pro-Tip……………….Some amazing replacement options

Day 45: Pro-Tip…..………………………………...Affirmation #9

Day 46: Favorite Resources…………………Use a food tracking app

Day 47: Favorite Resources………..*HealthyOut Healthy Meal Finder*

Day 48: Favorite Podcasts……………..*The Ultimate Health Podcast*

Day 49: Daily Challenge……………………………..Try carb cycling

Day 50: Favorite Resources………..Listen to your body + cut calories

Day 51: Daily Challenge…………………..Envision a long-term path

Day 52: Affirmations……………………………...…..…..Affirmation #10

Day 53: Daily Challenge…………Learning not to give into cravings

Day 54: Pro-Tip…………....…………….The most bang for your buck

Day 55: Success Story…………………………………………….Chaz Bono

Day 56: Affirmations……………………………...…..…..Affirmation #11

Progress Tracker……………………………………………….Check-In #5

Day 57: Pro-Tip…………………..Test removing foods for 1-2 weeks

Day 58: YouTube Alert!..……………………………………*Fit Men Cook*

Day 59: Success Story……………...…..…...……………….Jonah Hill

Day 60: Pro-Tip………………………...………..Ready for a new habit!?

Day 61: Daily Challenge…………………….Get someone on the wagon

Day 62: Pro-Tip…………..….……Make your cravings work for you

Day 63: Affirmations…………….…………...………..Affirmation #12

Day 64: Pro-Tip………………………….Physically change your state

Day 65: Success Story………………….…………..…John Goodman

Day 66: Congratulations!…………..…..……....…..Mama, I made it

Progress Tracker……………………………………………….Check-In #6